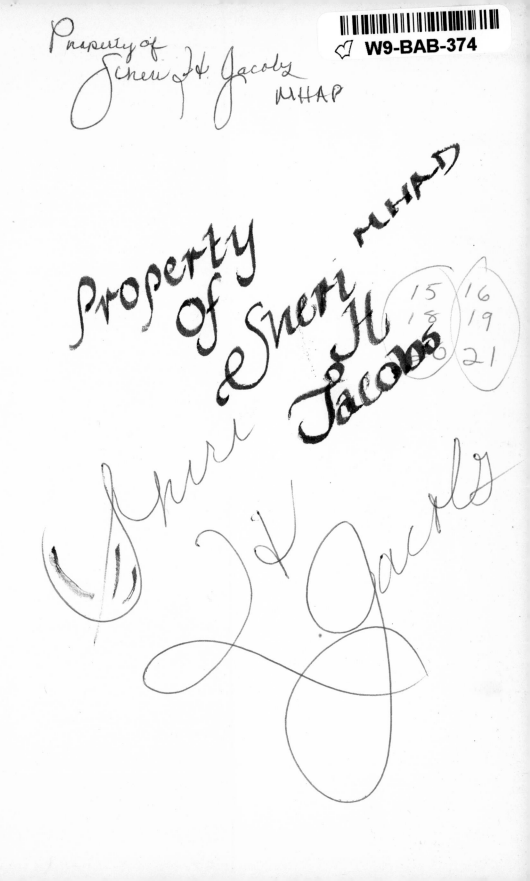

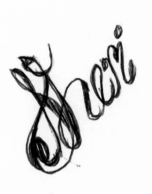

COUNSELLING AND THERAPY

An Introductory Survey

COUNSELLING AND THERAPY

An Introductory Survey

Sheri

Robert B. Burns
Chairman, School of Education
University of Bradford

1983 **MTP PRESS LIMITED**
a member of the KLUWER ACADEMIC PUBLISHERS GROUP
BOSTON / THE HAGUE / DORDRECHT / LANCASTER

Published in the UK and Europe by
MTP Press Limited
Falcon House
Lancaster, England

British Library Cataloguing in Publication Data

Burns, Robert B.
    Counselling and therapy.
    1. Counselling   2. Psychotherapy
    I. Title
    616.89'14   BF637.C6

    ISBN 0-85200-710-8

Published in the USA by
MTP Press
A division of Kluwer Boston Inc
190 Old Derby Street
Hingham, MA 02043, USA

Library of Congress Cataloging in Publication Data

Burns, R. B.
    Counselling and therapy.

    Bibliography: p.
    Includes index.
    1. Counseling.   2. Psychotherapy.   I. Title.
    [DNLM: 1. Psychotherapy.   2. Counseling.   WM 420 B967c]
    BF637.C6B83 1983   616.89'14   83-9379

    ISBN 0-85200-710-8

Printed in Great Britain by
Butler & Tanner Ltd, Frome and London

CONTENTS

FOREWORD

In discussing psychology and psychotherapy with students in both formal and informal settings, it has become obvious to me that many professionals and trainees in health, social service and education spheres often have misinformed, erroneous and often biased views of the aims, objectives and techniques involved in counselling and psychotherapy. There is a proliferation of therapies, some old, some new, which produce a confusing kaleidoscope of treatments on offer to a bewildered public.

The purpose of this text is to present in a relatively brief, objective form various current theories and practices in counselling or psychotherapy. This is difficult to do because brevity can itself bring about misunderstanding, misrepresentation or biased perception. The writer hopes that such has not occurred.

The text surveys the bewildering range of therapies available within and outside the Health, Social and Educational Services, to enable intelligent professionals in those services to be more aware of and sensitive to the treatments their clients are undergoing, may undergo or have undergone. Accounts of psychotherapeutic help are often buried in recondite journals, usually inaccessible to doctors, nurses, paramedics, social workers and teachers functioning at 'the coal face'. Few articles ever attempt a comprehensive survey or rapprochement; most simply argue for one therapy in a biased promotion.

The overall aim then is to acquaint the professional reader with the principal forms of therapy employed to alleviate personal emotional, social and educational difficulties, thereby enabling the professional to make decisions and recommendations about clients who may be undertaking one of a variety of therapies.

The purpose of the book is certainly not to teach readers how to become do-it-yourself therapists. It would be very dangerous for anyone to use the book in this way. Only formal training and practice under strict supervision can provide the necessary skills, knowledge and experience.

I would like to express my grateful thanks to my wife and family for their support and encouragement during the writing of this book. My gratitude also goes to my three typists, Eleanor Gordon, Margaret Butler and Helen Szutka.

Robert B. Burns
Gippsland Institute of Advanced Education
Victoria
Australia

Section I
INTRODUCTION

Chapter 1

SOME BACKGROUND AND ISSUES

HISTORICAL BACKGROUND TO PSYCHOTHERAPY

The early Chinese, Egyptians and Hebrews believed disordered behaviour was the result of possession by demons or evil spirits, and was to be exorcised by such techniques as incantation, magic and the use of herbal purgatives. If no improvement was effected more extreme measures were taken to ensure that the body would be an unpleasant dwelling place for the evil spirit. Flogging, starving, burning, even stoning to death were not infrequent forms of 'treatment'!

The first progress in the understanding of mental disorders came with the ideas of the Greek physician Hippocrates (c. 460–377 BC). Hippocrates rejected demonology, and maintained that behavioural disorder was the result of a disturbance in the balance of body fluids. He, and later Greek and Roman physicians, argued for a more humane treatment of the mentally ill. They stressed the importance of pleasant surroundings, exercise, proper diet, massage and soothing baths, as well as some less desirable methods, such as bleeding, purging and mechanical restraints. Although there were no institutions as such for the mentally ill, many individuals were cared for with great kindness by physicians in temples dedicated to the Greek and Roman gods.

This progress did not continue, however. During the Middle Ages, there was a revival of primitive superstition and demonology. The mentally ill were thought to be in league with the Devil and to possess supernatural powers with which they could cause floods, pestilence and injuries to others. People believed that by treating an insane person cruelly one was punishing the devil. This justified such measures as beating, starving and branding with hot irons. This type of cruelty culminated in the witchcraft trials that sentenced to death thousands of people (many of them mentally ill) between the fifteenth and seventeenth centuries.

3

In the latter part of the Middle Ages, asylums were created to cope with the mentally ill who roamed the streets. These were not treatment centres, but prisons with inmates chained in dark, filthy cells and treated more like animals than human beings. It was not until 1872, when Phillippe Pinel was put in charge of an asylum in Paris, that some improvement was made in the treatment of these unfortunate people. As an experiment, Pinel was allowed to remove the chains that restrained the inmates. Much to the amazement of the sceptics who thought he was mad to unchain such 'animals', Pinel's experiment was a success. When released from restraint, placed in clean and sunny rooms instead of dungeons, and treated kindly, many who had been considered hopelessly mad for years improved enough to leave the asylum.

Around the beginning of the twentieth century, great advances were made in medicine and psychology. The discovery of the syphilis spirochete in 1905 demonstrated that there was a physical cause for the mental disorder known as general paresis, and encouraged physicians who believed that mental illness was organic in origin. The work of Sigmund Freud and his followers laid the groundwork for an under-standing of mental illness as a function of psychological factors. Pavlov's laboratory experiments demonstrated that a state similar to an acute neurosis could be produced in animals by requiring them to make subtle discriminations beyond their capacities. Despite these scientific advances, the general public in the early 1900s still had no understanding of mental illness, and viewed mental hospitals and their inmates with fear and horror. The education of the public in the principles of mental health was begun through the efforts of Clifford Beers. As a young man Beers developed a manic–depressive psychosis and was hospitalized for 3 years in several American private and state hospitals. Although chains and other methods of torture had long since been abandoned, the straitjacket was still widely used to restrain excited patients. Lack of funds made the average mental hospital – with its overcrowded wards, poor food and un-sympathetic and frequently sadistic attendants – a far from pleasant place to live. After his recovery, Beers wrote about his experiences in a now-famous book, *A Mind That Found Itself* (1908), and this book did much to arouse public interest. Beers worked ceaselessly to educate the public in an understanding of mental illness.

During the past 20 years, emphasis has shifted from treating patients in hospitals to treating them within their home community whenever possible. Hospitalization, no matter how excellent the facilities, has inherent disadvantages. It cuts the patient off from family and friends. It tends to make the patient feel 'sick' and unable to cope with the outside world; it encourages dependency and may discourage active problem solving.

The demand for counselling and therapy seems to be increasing in the second half of this century. This may not imply that there are more neurotics, demoralized, or problem ridden persons around. It may reflect two things. Firstly, the former sources of solace, comfort and advice, the local priest, the family doctor, the closeknit family network may no longer be functioning in that way, as conventional religion has suffered a recession, as the personalized touch of the family doctor disappears in the bureaucracy of the health centre appointments book, and as the isolated nuclear family becomes the norm. Hence a new breed of professionals have emerged to fill the vacuum. Secondly, as knowledge of illness advances, medical practitioners are more aware that in many cases pills and potions are not the only cure or even the correct cure. Psychological rather than organic causes can be the real root of many headaches, tummy upsets, palpitations etc. *Mens sana in corpore sano* is recognized for its true worth now. Thus treatments involving therapy are recommended far more often, as a result of advances in knowledge in the art of healing the sick mind and its physical concomitants and behavioural manifestations.

A TROUBLE SHARED IS A TROUBLE HALVED

Man is a social animal; mutual co-operation and inter-dependence is the basis of the survival of the species whether the threat is a physical one such as famine or war, or whether it is psychological such as anxiety, stress and general unease. Psychotherapy is trouble sharing using a variety of non-verbal and verbal communicative techniques which can range from a sympathetic smile, through individual and group discussion to relaxation exercises. All human relationships can conceivably provide therapeutic 'medicine', involving conditions which allow the relief of distress in an ethos of support and understanding. Informal psychological aid can be provided by parents towards their children, by nurses towards their patients, by vicars towards their parishioners, by wives towards their husbands (and vice versa), by neighbour towards neighbour, by bar-tender towards a drunk, and by interest groups such as Gingerbread for one-parent families; just as formal support and assuaging of socio–psychological distress can be effected by social workers, psycho-therapists, clinical psychologists, school counsellors, marriage counsellors and the like. As the trouble is gradually revealed to and shared with another who creates a supportive accepting context, so catharsis may come about diminishing and hopefully extinguishing the trouble. All this sounds so simple, part of everyday good neighbourliness and good listening, so why is there the necessity to provide a book to explain therapeutic relationships and counselling? The answer is that there have developed a plethora of approaches and techniques derived from differing theoretical standpoints all presumably claiming to be the panacea for psychological distress. This book sets out to outline and explain these differences in approaches, and to consider their 'success' with different types of human problems.

It was argued above in a simple fashion that a therapeutic relationship may exist in any human interaction. However, psychotherapy is different from informal lay help in that the former is guided (even rigorously constrained) by particular theoretical bases which attempt in their own ways to explain the reasons for the clients' problems, and prescribe particular techniques for their alleviation. In all the psychotherapies there is an emphasis on the role of communication, with personal influence rather than surgical or medical offerings effecting beneficial change in the client. This is why the unfortunate bearer of psychological distress is referred to in this book as client rather than patient. While the personality of the professional person is vital in all medical and paramedical activities, nowhere is it more vital than in psychotherapy since the influence of the therapists in great measure determines the clients' attitudes towards the treatment, towards the therapist himself, and the expectations of a positive outcome.

COUNSELLING OR PSYCHOTHERAPY: THE SAME OR DIFFERENT?

Both these terms occur in the title of this book, because there is no strict agreement among authorities in the field as to whether counselling and psychotherapy connote the same set of process activities, or whether both terms must be maintained as there exist significant differences between the two. Many writers do regard counselling and psychotherapy as synonymous. For example, Brammer and Shostrom (1964) view counselling and psychotherapy from the standpoint of therapeutic psychology:

> Therapeutic psychology applied through counselling and psycho-
> therapy is primarily a process of building understanding, integrating
> disparate elements of the personality, and enabling the client to utilise
> his good judgement, social skills, problem-solving and planning
> abilities.

Patterson (1973) emphasizes the professional status of the counsellor, but does not distinguish his role from the psychotherapist's:

> Counselling (or psychotherapy) is a relationship, involving verbal interaction, between a professionally trained person and an individual or group of individuals voluntarily seeking help with a problem which is psychological in nature, for the purpose of effecting a change in the individuals seeking help.

The simplest definition of both was offered by Truax and Carkhuff (1967). They claim:

> Counselling or psychotherapy is aimed at producing constructive behavioural and personality change. The beauty of this definition is that it can embrace all the different theoretical allegiances and methods of practice without offending any.

So definitions of counselling and therapy tend to be synonymous, and in many definitions and discussions the two terms are lumped together. There is little doubt that counselling and psychotherapy are both processes involving a special kind of relationship between a person who is trained to provide help (the counsellor or therapist) and a person who is seeking help with a psychological problem (the client). Nelson-Jones (1982) claims that the nature of the relationship is essentially the same, if not identical, in both counselling and psychotherapy. The process that occurs also does not seem to differ from one to the other. Nor do there seem to be any distinct techniques or group of techniques that separate counselling and psychotherapy.

Halmos (1965) writes:

> Basically and essentially all the practitioners have a common origin and aim; their common ancestor is the giver of spiritual solace and their common aim is health, sanity, a state of unspecified virtue, even a state of grace, or merely a return to the virtues of the community, adjustment.

The personality and learning theories that underlie many counselling and psychotherapy approaches and techniques are the same. In fact it is difficult to distinguish between theories of learning, theories of personality, and theories of counselling or psychotherapy. All are concerned with behaviour, and are thus theories of behaviour. Moreover, the same approach may be labelled as a therapy in one text and as a form of counselling in another. This dual naming occurs notably with Rogers' Client Centred Therapy or Counselling.

Even the objectives of counselling and therapy are similar. The objectives of counselling have been identified by the Committee on Definition, Division of Counseling Psychology of the American Psychological Association, as 'to help individuals toward overcoming obstacles to their personal growth, wherever these may be encountered, and toward achieving optimum development of their personal resources'. Most psychotherapists would accept these as goals of psychotherapy also. However, Tyler (1969) believes that counselling is not aimed at repairing damage done to the client in the past, to stimulate inadequate development of some stunted aspect of his personality, but is the process of helping a person attain a clear sense of personal identity, along with acceptance of limitations. Again, it would appear that many would reject these restrictions on counselling and would accept as a goal of counselling the goal of psychotherapy, which according to Tyler is aimed at change in developmental structure. Another distinction advanced by Tyler (1969) is that counselling is performed on 'normal' persons whose problems are concerned with developing their potential, whereas psychotherapy concerns clients who are deficient in some respect. This leads to a distinction between counselling and therapy in terms of severity of disturbance. There is of course no sharp dividing line that can be drawn here. But the implication is that when a client has a serious psychological disturbance or is handicapped in functioning 'normally' because of such a disturbance, the process is called 'psychotherapy', as it is seen as a remedial process to bring the individual up to 'normal'. When a client is not seriously disturbed but rather has the problems of the so-called normal person, which interfere with the development of the individual's potential, then the process is called 'counselling'. But even accepting this criterion of disturbance, counsellors practice psychotherapy, while psychotherapists practice counselling; for it is clear that a therapist cannot and does not make a determination that the client, after a period of psychotherapy, is now functioning at a minimal 'normal' level and should therefore be transferred to a counsellor for help beyond this point. Other writers argue too that counselling and psychotherapy are a continuum of services that parallel both a continuum of disturbance, and a continuum of treatment depth. For instance Vance and Volsky (1962), suggest that counselling deals with so-called normal individuals whose problems are developmental in nature, whereas psychotherapy is concerned with those who are in some way deficient. Their continuum is based on the kind of people with whom the two services work. Counselling is largely concerned with the so-called normal individual and is characterized by terms such as 'conscious awareness, 'problem solving', 'education', 'supportive', and 'situational'; psychotherapy, on the other hand, is concerned with reconstruction, depth emphasis, analysis, and focusing on the unconscious, and especially on neurotic and emotional problems. Psychotherapists tend to look for what is wrong and how to treat it, while counselling psychologists tend to look for what is right and how to use it.

A special committee of the American Psychological Association suggested that counselling involves helping individuals plan for a productive role in their social environments. 'Whether the person being helped with such planning is sick or well, abnormal or normal, is really irrelevant. The focus is on assets, skills, strengths, and possibilities for further development. Personality difficulties are strengths and possibilities for further development. Personality difficulties are dealt with only when they constitute obstacles to the individual's forward progress' (APA Report 1961, p. 6). Hence, the focus of the APA continuum is not the individual, but the manner in which the counsellor and psychotherapist work with their respective clients. Wolberg (1954) attempted to differentiate counselling from psychotherapy by defining three kinds of approaches: supportive, insight–reeducative, and insight–reconstructive. He considered the first two approaches appropriate for counsellors and the third for psychotherapists. As with other attempts to delineate function, Wolberg appeared to regard counselling and psychotherapy as elements of a continuum. According to English and English (1958, p. 127), 'While usually applied to help the normal counselee, counselling merges by imperceptible degrees into psychotherapy'.

Let us concede that counselling and psychotherapy indeed exist along a continuum, as depth of treatment, yet they are related ways of helping people in need. At one end of the continuum are intrapersonal conflicts; at the other are conflicts that involve role definitions.

Most psychotherapy occurs in the area of intrapersonal conflict of high intensity. The counsellor works at the other end of that continuum with people who are more likely to respond to short-term, more direct kinds of learning experiences. The difference then is that counselling works towards helping people to understand and develop their personality in relation to specific role problems; psychotherapy aims at reorganization of the personality through interaction with a therapist.

Counselling does not attempt to restructure personality, but to develop what already exists. It is chiefly concerned with individuals' adjustments to themselves, to significant others in their lives and to the cultural environment in which they find themselves, but the various activities associated with counselling and psychotherapy share enough common ground to warrant considering them together. Although marriage-guidance counsellors and school counsellors, for instance, may wish to distinguish their role very clearly from that of a psychoanalyst or clinical psychologist, such differing roles and emphases often seem to obscure how much those who work with people have in common, particularly when one looks at the principles, aims and ethics of the various offerings.

It is apparent that most authorities on counselling and therapy who either practice, write and/or research in the area find it difficult to distinguish clearly between the roles of various professionals involved in such helping services. Henceforth in this book the single term *therapist* shall be used to refer to any person who functions professionally in a therapeutic context to bring about more adaptive behaviour in a person or persons seeking help. The term *client* will be used generally for the person seeking help. This avoids the medical or illness connotation which surrounds the term 'patient'.

So it is not possible to make any clear distinction between counselling and psychotherapy save in terms of depth of exploration. Such a classification has been offered by Cawley (1977). His types 1–3 (Figure 1) involve increasing depths of exploration. Psychotherapy 1 is what any good doctor, teacher or other professional does. It involves an awareness of the person and his problem, and requires an ability to communicate and empathize with people from different backgrounds. The doctor decides to refer a patient to a psychiatrist or psychotherapist, or the teacher arranges for a pupil to see the school counsellor. Temporary help is given for the problem and apprehension about the impending visit to the professional is allayed.

Psychotherapy 2 is what a good therapist (or social worker) does. It encompasses Psychotherapy 1, but requires ability to understand and communicate with clients suffering from a range of psychological disturbance.

Psychotherapy 3 would be what many people mean by psychoanalysis. It includes the characteristics of Psychotherapies 1 and 2 which relate to the therapist's attitude to the client – respect, understanding and acceptance. Dynamic psychoanalysis makes the doctor–client relation-ship its focus, and uses Freudian psychodynamic principles to explore and understand clients' problems. Transference phenomena are encouraged since they throw light on the continuing influence of past relationships, from which the client can begin to free himself as he comes to recognize them.

Psychotherapy 4 (in Cawley's classification) is behavioural psycho-

	Level 1	Level 2	Level 3
Type of Therapy	Supportive Therapy and Counselling for usually healthy persons in times of crisis, e.g. job loss, bereavement	Psychotherapy to facilitate self awareness and self understanding	Psychoanalysis and related depth approaches
Given by	Student counsellors, doctors, marriage guidance counsellors, etc	Non-psychoanalytic psycho-therapists, e.g. Rogerian, existential, Gestalt	Freudian oriented analysts
Aims and themes	Non-directive and client centred unburdening of problems to sympathetic listener ventilation of feelings within supportive relationship discussion of current problems with non-judgemental helper Advice and reassurance Limited aims	clarification of problems, their nature and origins, within a deepening relationship	confrontation of defences interpretation of unconscious motives and transference phenomena repetition, remembering and reconstruction of past regression to less adult and less rational functioning resolution of conflicts by re-experiencing and working them through

Depth of exploration

Cawley's levels

therapy. It uses techniques of behaviour modification based on learning theory. These methods are developed and used largely by clinical psychologists, but psychiatrists and psychiatric nurses are also being trained in their use. Because its practitioners wish to be scientific, in the sense of measuring and validating, Psychotherapy 4 tends to concern itself with the patient's manifest behaviour, being more easily quantified than inner experience which at best can only be partially expressed in the other approaches. Symptoms are regarded as maladaptive patterns of behaviour or 'bad habits', learned as a result of past experience and not corrected. Behaviour therapy aims at correction of the maladaptive behaviour.

For each of the therapies outlined in this book the general procedure will be to identify the therapy in terms of its rationale, core concepts, goals and other essential elements. Then follows a consideration of the techniques or implementation methods. Finally a general evaluation concludes the discussion.

The evaluations are not thorough critiques of the theories, but rather summaries of the major contributions of each approach and consideration of some of the major objections or criticisms that have been or might be raised against them.

The presentations are intended to be descriptive rather than polemic. There is no attempt to argue in favour of one approach above all others, only to provide indications of the range of applications for which each is most suitable. The final chapter provides an evaluative comparison of effectiveness, but this is done not out of any attempt to denigrate or eulogize particular approaches. It is simply an attempt to show how difficult it is to demonstrate the comparative effectiveness of various therapies.

SHARED THERAPEUTIC FUNCTIONS OF THE RATIONALES AND PROCEDURES OF PSYCHOTHERAPY

Despite marked differences in content, all rationales and procedures in psychotherapy, reinforced by the setting, share six therapeutic functions:

(1) They strengthen the therapeutic relationship. Since the therapist represents the majority society, his mere acceptance of the client as worthy of help reduces the latter's sense of isolation and re-establishes his sense of contact with his group. This is further reinforced by the fact that therapist and client adhere to the same belief system (Frank, 1977), a powerful unifying force in all groups. Explanations of the client's symptoms or problems in terms of a theory of therapy,

implicitly convey to him that he is not unique, since the rationale obviously must have developed out of experiences with many clients. The treatment procedure also serves as a vehicle for maintaining the therapist–client relationship over stretches when little seems to be happening, by giving both participants work to do.

(2) They provide hope. This keeps him coming but is a powerful healing force in itself (Frank, 1968). Hope is sustained by being translated into concrete expectations.

(3) They provide cognitive and experiential learning by offering him new information about his problems and possible ways of dealing with them, or new ways of conceptualizing what he already knows. All schools of psychotherapy agree that intellectual insight is not sufficient to produce change.

(4) They provide a sense of mastery. Ability to control one's environment starts with the ability to accept and master one's own impulses and feelings, an achievement which in itself overcomes anxiety and strengthens self-confidence. A powerful source of a sense of mastery is being able to name and order one's experiences, a function facilitated by one of the therapeutic rationales. The sense of mastery is reinforced by success experiences, which all therapeutic procedures provide in one form or another. These successes maintain the client's hopes, increase his sense of mastery over his feelings and behaviour, and reduce his fear of failure. The role of success experiences is most obvious in behaviour therapy, which is structured to provide continual evidence of progress and aims to have every session end with a sense of attainment.

In short, evidence available to date strongly suggests that in treating most conditions for which persons come or are brought into psychotherapy, the shared functions of different rationales and procedures, not their differing content, contribute most of the therapeutic power. These functions, which are interwoven, all help to re-establish the client's morale by combating his sense of isolation, re-awakening his hopes, supplying him with new information as a basis for both cognitive and experiential learning, stirring him emotionally, providing experiences of mastery and success, and encouraging him to apply what he has learned. The general aim of all the many psychotherapies is personal psychological growth, so that each client is able to satisfy his human needs for acceptance, (by self and other), recognition, affection, mastery of the environment and positive self feeling (self concept) through the modification and/or removal of maladaptive emotions, behaviour, attitudes and feelings. One person cannot take a plane trip because he is afraid; another person cannot stop thinking certain thoughts that make her profoundly uncomfortable; another person is always too 'down' to function optimally, and another person finds it difficult to speak and interact with others. In all cases, behaviour that the client seems unable to control appears to direct him or her in ways that create unhappiness. Psychotherapy then attempts to aid the patient become more competent in pursuing life goals, and thereby happier by stimulating mastery over the thoughts, feelings and actions that hinder this competence. Where the therapies diverge is over (1) whether they are oriented towards present difficulties, towards past problems or towards new potentialities in the future, (2) whether they focus on external behaviour or internal conflicts below the level of conscious awareness, (3) whether they focus on the client himself or on the client functioning within pathogenic forces of his social environment, (4) whether they concentrate on verbal or non-verbal interactions, (5) whether they are directive or non-directive, or (6) whether they seek emotional or intellectual insight. Such variety exists because the underlying theoretical rationales differ (i.e. a variety of personality and learning theories underpin the procedures). Additionally, it is possible to discern strands of social, cultural, philosophic and historical influences weaving their variety of orientation into the multi-coloured dream coat of therapeutic procedures.

It is possible on the basis of these differing emphases, influences and foci to categorize a multitude of competing and often mutually antagonistic therapies into three general groups. These groupings which act to give structure to this book are:

(1) *Dynamic psychoanalytically derived therapies*
   The roots of the dynamic school of therapy are found in the psychoanalytic theory and work of Sigmund Freud. The dynamic school emphasizes the thoughts, feelings and past life of the client, particularly unconscious ones, and the need for insight into them. Dynamic therapists see the internal conflicts as arising from traumatic experiences in early life and seek to unearth their sources and thereby resolve them.

(2) *Behaviourist approaches*
   The behaviour therapies have their basis in the learning theories and work of such as Pavlov, Watson, Thorndike, Skinner, Bandura and others. Concentrating their techniques mainly on the specific overt actions of the client, the behaviour therapies differ from others, which regard such behaviour as only symptomatic. Using techniques

derived largely from principles of learning discovered in the psychological laboratory, behaviour therapists attempt to bring about
change by modifying these actions in a more adaptive way.
Behaviour therapists believe that the client's ability to overcome
specific symptoms will promote more general improvement by
enhancing his social competence and self-confidence. Hence they
attempt to tailor their methods to combat the client's specific
complaints and, have succeeded to some extent with complaints
which are fairly circumscribed.

(3) *Humanistic approaches*
The humanistic therapies are much more diverse, and have their
basic foundation in a phenomenological view of man. Emphasizing
the unique qualities of each individual client's vision of himself in the
various life settings, the humanistic techniques are quite varied.
Typically, they range from the relational and insight-oriented
techniques used by existential analysts (similar to dynamic therapies)
through the Rogerian client-centred approach to the directive
rational-emotive techniques used by Albert Ellis (claimed by some to
be behavioural techniques). They all emphasize helping the patient to
open up the future – that is, to discover new potentialities for personal
satisfaction and growth.

The proliferation of therapeutic approaches is such that the same problem
can be treated in a variety of ways. For example:

Mary is a teenager with a severe stuttering problem. She sees a therapist
who might approach her problem in one of many ways.

e.g. Psychoanalyst
      The therapist assumes that the stuttering behaviour is an
      expression of an unconscious conflict associated with hostility,
      particularly toward Mary's parents. Therapy would involve
      trying to bring into awareness this underlying conflict through
      the interpretation of free association, dreams, slips of the
      tongue and repressed memories.

or   Behaviour Modifier
      The therapist explores the possibility that the stuttering
      behaviour was a classically conditioned response. Techniques
      to treat stuttering might involve negative practice, a technique
      requiring a person to stutter repeatedly on purpose. Rhythmic
      speech patterns and operant conditioning involving rewards

for appropriate speech might also be used. Finally, if stuttering increases as anxiety increases, then relaxation training might be used.

Peter is a compulsive eater. He weighs 252 pounds. Seeking help from a professional therapist he might be treated in one of a variety of ways:

e.g. Psychoanalyst
      The therapist explores early childhood memories, the content of dreams, free association and slips of the tongue to determine the symbolic meaning of the eating behaviour. The psychoanalyst would look for the possibility that Peter is symbolically expressing strong needs for love and aggression.

or   Behaviour Modifier
      The therapist explores the rewarding aspects of overeating and determines whether such behaviour allows Peter to avoid other anxiety-evoking situations. The therapist may set up a conditioning form of treatment in which Peter is punished for overeating or thinking about eating, or is rewarded for non-eating behaviour. The therapist might try to increase behaviour incompatible with eating or change Peter's eating patterns. If eating leads to anxiety reduction, relaxation techniques may be used to lower anxiety levels.

or   Client-Centred Therapist
      In both cases, stuttering and overeating, the therapist makes no assumption about the underlying meaning of symptomatic behaviour. Therapy would focus on helping the client clarify values, goals and feelings. The client would be helped in understanding how he or she feels, and would be led to a non-judgemental accepting atmosphere to experience those feelings in the here and now.

TWO CONTEMPORARY ISSUES

Currently there are several important issues facing psychotherapy. The first is clients' rights, which is a two fold concern for the civil liberties of persons whose behaviour society labels as deviant, and who are behaviourally modified (manipulated?) into conforming with some imposed societal norm, and for the plight of involuntary hospitalized mental patients.

Clients' rights

Szasz (1960), a psychiatrist who is highly critical of psychotherapy, gave this movement its intellectual impetus by claiming that mental illness is a 'myth'. He believes that to conceptualize maladaptive behaviour as an 'illness' is to use a dangerous metaphor because it authorizes, in pseudo-scientific guise, the moral labelling and social control of deviant individuals. Although the alleged goal of this labelling and control is benevolent paternalism, for Szasz the only behaviour that authorizes unwanted state intrusion into a person's life is the commission of a crime. Any other intrusion is an impermissible infringement on personal liberty. If a person shows certain abnormal behaviour – for example, a phobia of crowds, compulsive rituals or mute unresponsiveness, are these 'maladaptive habits', or are they 'symptoms of an underlying disorder'? This is an issue on which therapists disagree. Behaviour therapists say, 'Change the behaviour and you have cured the disorder'. Psychoanalysts and other more traditional therapists maintain that maladaptive behaviour is only a symptom of an underlying 'disease'. They view mental disorders as analogous to physical disorders, and consider it futile to treat the symptoms without removing the underlying pathology. (The physician treating a case of syphilis does not simply apply an ointment to the rash but destroys the syphilis spirochete with antibiotics.) According to this view, a phobia or other neurotic symptom is only the surface expression of more complex emotional difficulties; removal of the phobia without treatment of the underlying problem may result in symptom substitution. The client develops new symptoms (new neurotic defences against the anxiety caused by internal conflict) if the therapist eliminates the original symptom without curing the underlying conflict; just as a weed will pop out at a nearby spot if the gardener only pulls off the stalk but leaves the root in the ground. Behaviour therapy is criticized by some as being a superficial method of treatment that removes the symptoms without dealing with the inner conflicts, thereby leaving the patient vulnerable to symptom substitution.

Behaviour therapists, of course, disagree. They maintain that there need be no underlying conflict. A neurosis is a set of maladaptive habits formed through the process of conditioning; once the habits (symptoms) are extinguished and replaced by more adaptive ones, the 'illness is cured'. The symptom *is* the problem, and eliminating the symptom eliminates the problem. The debate is not easily settled, for a number of reasons; but the evidence suggests that symptom substitution does not occur very often. Several reviews of post-treatment evaluation studies found few instances of new symptoms up to 2 years after successful treatment by behaviour modification methods (Paul and Bernstein, 1973). Instead, the removal of a disturbing 'symptom' usually creates better emotional health; the person's self-esteem is increased by this accomplishment, and other people respond more favourably to the individual once his or her behaviour has changed.

The broader issue of whether abnormal behaviour should be viewed as 'mental illness' or 'maladaptive behaviour' is more difficult to resolve. There does seem to be some advantage in minimizing the disease concept, at least as far as neuroses are concerned, and focusing instead on the very practical problem of how people can change their behaviour to cope more satisfactorily with the problems of life. One psychiatrist sums up the issue in this way: 'Our adversaries are not demons, witches, fate or mental illness. We have no enemy whom we can fight, exorcise; or dispel by 'cure'. What we do have are problems in *living* – whether these be biologic, economic, political, or sociopsychological' (Szasz, 1967, p. 118).

The consequence of using a psychological model rather than a medical disease model is that the people who seek assistance, are no longer regarded by themselves and by others as psychiatric patients, and will be expected by themselves and others to play a more active part in overcoming their difficulties. The significance of this change is conveyed, in part by replacing the term *patient* by the term *client*. Even the term client with its connotations of the legal and business world is not totally satisfactory; it too conveys a stiff, starchy and distant impression of personal relationships.

On the other hand, to completely deny that any illness is involved in serious mental disorders does not seem fully justified. Current research makes the complex interplay between 'physical' and 'mental' functioning increasingly clear. To view psychotic disorders as solely a problem of re-education is a misleading oversimplification. Biochemical abnormalities can play an important role in schizophrenia and in some depressive disorders. Psychotherapists are now faced with at least two important questions: first, when is the involuntary application of psychotherapy to an unwilling client justified; and second, when is the label of mental illness used to mask a therapist's social value preference. In other words, can such categorization lead to harmful labelling of the client and to therapy that fosters the therapist's value preferences rather than the client's autonomy?

An example that raises both questions involves the rights and treatment of homosexual patients. Davison (1976) a behaviour therapist, is concerned with the coercive force exerted on homosexuals to begin treatment. He believes, as most therapists do, that the patient must enter therapy voluntarily. The treatment of a client forced into a therapeutic situation, whether by law or by private pressures, raises ethical issues for the potential therapist. For instance, granted a persons' unwillingness to change, we may ask if such measures unduly infringe on the dignity of the individual.

Regarding homosexual behaviour, social pressures, insidious and otherwise, may be a primary motivating force for the homosexual's desire to change sexual orientation. Davison suggests that all therapies aimed at changing the sexual orientation of homosexuals be stopped, even with voluntary patients, because the existence of any therapeutic programme lends credence to the view that homosexuality in itself is pathological, which Davison does not believe.

Is psychotherapy sexist?

The second area of concern is the question of women and psychotherapy. Some practitioners and some members of the women's movement feel that the theory and practice of psychotherapy are sexist (e.g. Chesler, 1972). They see psychotherapy as a repressive force narrowing the options of women clients instead of allowing them a greater diversity in their lives. As in the treatment of homosexuals, the therapist's values play a major role in what he or she sees as the goal of treatment for the client, namely, what behaviour should be changed through therapy. How should a therapist treat a woman client who, because of social pressure, has been made, first, to feel uncomfortable with a non-traditional female role, and second, to seek therapy promoting conformity to the traditional female role? Similarly, should the focus of treatment for an unhappily married client ever be an acceptance of traditional marital roles, even if such treatment would ameliorate the immediate marital tensions?

Many women presently feel that they can receive more understanding and less prejudicial treatment from a female therapist. Some women's organizations have approved lists of therapists, both male and female, who they feel have a positive, less stereotyped orientation toward female patients, seeing women as active and striving for themselves. Therapeutic programmes presently are being developed to deal with problems that especially confront women in our society. Some of these, such as the work being done on assertiveness, are in direct conflict with stereotyped views of women. Even with such therapies, however, the psychotherapist has to decide when and with whom to use these techniques.

This opening chapter has attempted to introduce the problems of trying to differentiate between the twin processes of counselling and therapy, and to provide a brief overview of some major approaches to counselling and guidance. It would seem (1) that counselling and psychotherapy differ only in their depth of treatment, (2) that the various major approaches differ in their views of the courses of disordered behaviour and their philosophic perspective of mankind, and (3) that problems of clients' rights, accusations of manipulation, the dignity of the individual and illness connotations of maladaptive behaviour permeate all approaches of treatment to a greater or lesser extent.

Further reading

Beers, C. (1908). *A Mind That Found Itself*. (New York: Doubleday)

Brammer, L. M. and Shostrum, E. L. (1977). *Therapeutic Psychology*. (Englewood Cliffs: Prentice-Hall)

Carkhuff, R. (1969). *Helping and Human Relations. Vol. 1 & 2*. (New York: Holt, Rinehart and Winston)

Frank, J. D. (1973). *Persuasion & Healing*. (London: Johns Hopkins University Press)

Halmos, P. (1965). *The Faith of the Counsellor*. (London: Constable)

Tyler, L. (1969). *The Work of the Counselor*. (New York: Appleton-Century-Crofts)

Szasz, T. S. (1960). *The Myth of Mental Illness*. (New York: Harper Row)

Section II
PSYCHOANALYTIC APPROACHES

Chapter 2

PSYCHOANALYSIS

Psychoanalysis is both a set of theories and a therapy produced by Freud's genius. Freud's written output was prolific; the standard edition of his collected works runs to twenty-four volumes. From 1895 when he first began to publish his ideas on psychoanalysis, until his death in 1939, he developed his theory in a variety of directions. Not surprisingly his views changed during this time in response to new evidence and to new clinical thoughts and discussions with his colleagues (though some would say that he remained remarkably impervious to criticism). For these reasons it is difficult to adequately summarize his approach in the space available here. What will be attempted is to introduce the main tenets of his theory.

Freud lived during a creative period in the history of science. Darwin, Einstein, Mendeleylev (but to mention a few) were exciting the world with their new notions. Freud's genius was to take up some of these notions and create a view of man as an energy system. He applied laws of dynamics to man's personality, creating a dynamic psychology, studying the transformations and exchanges of energy within the personality. A neurologist, he was also influenced by the materialistic, laissez-faire, competitive philosophy of the era, and so had a biological mechanical approach rather than social approach to man. He saw human relationships as an 'economic' relationship, buying and selling oneself, creating a market, using others as a means to an end. Man basically was selfish.

After training as a doctor, he specialized in the treatment of nervous disorders. He became interested in the use of hypnosis in treatment and studied with Charcot in Paris, but became dissatisfied with the outcome of this technique. He then became interested in Joseph Breuer's development of the cathartic form of therapy, in which clients related the details of their symptoms and when they occurred while the doctor listened. Freud adopted and developed this 'talking out' technique and it was upon this technique and the free associations of his clients – the recounting of everything, no matter how ridiculous and apparently irrelevant, that comes into consciousness – that he began to build his dynamic theory.

THE THEORY

Basic tenets of the theory

The role of the unconscious

The concept of the unconscious is central to psychoanalytic theory. Freud believed that most of our motives are unconscious, and that unconscious motivation, in some degree, affects every aspect of our behaviour, from the profession we choose to the clothes we wear, to whether or not we smoke cigarettes. What Freud did was to develop a conception of the unconscious as the source of the mental energy, or dynamism, which is the driving force of behaviour.

Freud's predecessors had conceived of the unconscious as a waste paper basket for ideas and memories which are no longer important to the individual, and thus drift out of conscious awareness. Freud, on the other hand, viewed the unconscious as a dynamic force. He believed that the material in the unconscious is mostly disturbing in nature and requires the expenditure of mental energy to prevent it from forcing itself into consciousness; such material can only reach awareness by devious means such as in dreams.

Psychological determinism

This conception of a dynamic unconscious full of energy or psyche leads to the doctrine of psychological determinism, wherein everything we say or do, including slips of the tongue, free associations, and dreams, reflects some unconscious motivation. For a Freudian, nothing happens by chance. There is a psychological reason for everything. Freud regarded no aspect of human behaviour as accidental.

In his early work with hysterical patients Freud showed that their apparently irrational symptoms could be explained in terms of the repression of painful memories. This does not mean that Freud denied the existence of events which are accidental, i.e. which are brought about by objects and forces outside the control of the individual who experiences them. If you are involved in a car accident, it may well not be the direct result of your own behaviour but may be due to another road user or the condition of the road surface, or any other factor outside your control. On the other hand, if you are regularly involved in motor accidents (above the national norm) then there might be a case for arguing that psychological factors are playing a part in your poor driving behaviour. Freud argues that many instances of so-called accidental behaviour have psychological determinants which can be identified, particularly if the accidents occur frequently.

Freud's notion of psychological determinism does not state that each aspect of behaviour has one single cause. On the contrary, Freud believed in the principle of overdetermination, or multiple determination, according to which every psychic event is determined by the simultaneous action of several different causes.

Goal-directed dynamics

This principle asserts that all behaviour is motivated and goal-directed. Even apathy can be conceived of as goal-directed. For Freud, apathy is one way in which an individual defends certain aspects of his personality against disturbing thoughts or emotions by showing little interest in anything which might prove threatening.

The idea that behaviour is goal-directed is common to most approaches within psychology, although in different ways. But this idea was undeniably enhanced by the psychoanalyst's deliberate habit of looking for the goal underlying an individual's behaviour. According to Freud the symbolic content of a dream is imbued with wish-fulfilment. Although the idea of a purposeful behaviour is not unique to the psychodynamic approach, the goal-directed nature of the unconscious is an original Freudian concept.

Developmental approach

Underlying this approach is the belief that an individual's behaviour is greatly influenced by prior experience. In particular, adult behaviour is the product of the experience of the growing child. Although Freud placed great emphasis on the power of instinctual needs (such as hunger, thirst and sex) in motivating behaviour, he did not believe that the development of a person was totally governed by instinctual and biological factors. Rather, the complex attributes of the adult are determined through interaction with the physical and social environment. For this reason it is essential to look at the longitudinal growth of an individual's personality in attempting to explain his present behaviour.

According to Freud, a child's first experiences have a powerful influence on later behaviour through moulding the pliable mind to form the foundations on which the adult personality is built. Based on this reasoning, the psychodynamic approach places great significance on the experiences of childhood, and in particular, on the resolution of conflicts which arise during the first 5 years of life. The psychoanalytic movement was the first psychological discipline to give such emphasis to the early period of life.

Structure of personality

Freud describes the psychical apparatus which underlies human behaviour as consisting of three structural components: the *id*, *ego* and *superego*. They are abstract concepts which derive their meaning within the psychoanalytic explanation of behaviour. Freud's model is built out of abstract components which relate to the forces governing behaviour. The id is the source of all mental energy and provides the driving force of behaviour, driving all behaviour in the direction of immediate gratification of the individual's biological needs – hunger, thirst, sex, etc.

As the individual interacts with his environment so some of the id energy changes into ego. The ego functions to maintain the individual as a whole, while at the same time adapting to external reality as it learns to relate external stimuli to its own needs. The functions of the ego are always directed towards external reality and so include psychological functions such as memory, perception, language, thinking, learning, motor skills and action.

Whereas the id represents the demands generated within the individual, the superego represents the internalization of the demands normally generated outside the individual by his culture or society. These demands are initially communicated to the child through the dictates of the parents and form the two sub-structures of the ego ideal, the child's conception of the behaviour of which his parents approve, and conscience, the child's conception of the behaviour his parents will condemn as morally bad. It is as if the parents were inside the child's head waiting to make demands of his behaviour whenever id impulses arise which do not conform with the norms of society. Freud's theory thus places great emphasis on the influence and learning of parental attitudes in the formation of the child's personality.

The psyche also has different qualities or levels, the conscious, preconscious and unconscious. The id is totally unconscious whereas the other two structures span the unconscious–preconscious–conscious distinction. Freud considers, rather tentatively, that there are two basic instinctive forces stemming from the id, Eros, the love instinct, the energy of which is referred to as 'libido'; and the destructive or death instinct (Thanatos).

The dynamics of personality are based on the notion of conflict. The structural components of personality, the id, ego and superego, together with the external forces acting on an individual, interact in such a way as to be in continual conflict. These conflicts require resolution in order for a person to function normally. The ego for example has three harsh masters: the id, the superego and external reality. The id is always governed by the pleasure principle and makes demands on the ego for the immediate gratification of its instinctual needs. The ego has somehow to modify these demands in line with the restrictions imposed on it by the superego. At the same time, the ego has to consider the id's demands in terms of the possibilities presented by external reality, thereby functioning in accordance with the reality principle. The ego's job is to co-ordinate the demands of the id and the restrictions of the superego and external reality. It is the ego which has to find all the compromises because its masters are not interested in compromising; they demand full obedience.

The main product of these mental conflicts is the experience of anxiety. This is manifested within the ego. A different form of anxiety is associated with each of the three masters of the ego: neurotic anxiety with the id, moral anxiety with the superego, and objective anxiety with external reality. The ego attempts to reduce anxiety by resolving the conflict through the co-ordination of internal and external forces.

The well adjusted person is governed by his ego; the anxious neurotic by guilt stemming from his superego; the psychopath by his id. The aim of psychoanalysis is to restore the balance. 'Where id was, there shall ego be' (Freud, 1933).

If the ego is unable to resolve a particular conflict then it resorts to protecting itself from the ensuing anxiety by various strategies known as defence mechanisms. The most commonly employed mechanism is repression, by which the impulses from the id which create the conflict are shut out of awareness by the ego. Freud (1926) suggested nine varieties of defence mechanism. Later analysts have extended this part of his model, e.g. Anna Freud (1936). The ego defences usually operate at an unconscious level counteracting impulses arising at the same level. Defence mechanisms are not necessarily unhealthy; indeed they are a necessary process within a normally functioning personality. Although these processes may prove inadequate in the long term, they provide the ego with a means of short term control over inner conflicts and anxiety.

Psychosexual stages

The different stages of psychosexual development in childhood represent the redistribution of libido from one erogenous zone, mouth (oral), anus (anal), phallus (phallic), or genitals (genital) to another. Although in Freud's model these stages are not entirely separate nor is a phase ever entirely left behind, the approximate periods of their major importance are:

oral stage   – birth to 2 years   0 - 2
anal stage   – 2 years to 4/5 years 2 - 5
phallic stage – 4/5 years to 7 years 5 - 7
latency stage – 7 years to puberty   7 - 12
genital stage – puberty

At each stage of development one cathects or concentrates on the part of the body that defines that stage. No strong libidinal cathexis is ever completely dissolved, and people retain cathexes that were more appropriate to earlier periods in their lives. These 'immature' cathexes are known as fixations. Fixations are primarily unconscious and are a general feature of psychosexual development – everyone has fixations of some kind. The complementary concept is regression – the return to an earlier mode or object of gratification, i.e. one regresses to an earlier fixation. Fixations result from either excessive gratification or undue frustration of a particular mode of satisfaction. In addition to determining the kinds of satisfactions a person will seek, fixations give a distinctive flavour to a person's interpersonal style. For example, excessive deprivation at the oral stage may result in an 'oral-dependent' personality, a longing for maternal support that manifests itself as passivity, low self-esteem, and indulgence in such 'oral' activities as drinking, smoking, eating and nail-biting. Excessive oral gratification can produce an 'oral-aggressive' personality characterized by a self-confident, quarrelsome, verbal aggressiveness (symbolic biting of the mother's breast).

Children who experience rigid toilet training, according to Freud, may develop severe anxiety about fecal matter. This sometimes results in a fixation at the anal stage and an 'anti-retentive' personality. Such people are stingy, pedantic, fussy about rules, compulsively neat and tidy, and overly concerned with the functioning of their bowels. Children who, on the other hand, undergo leisurely toilet training may as adults spend money freely, ignore rules, and appear slovenly in their personal habits; they are not anxious about fecal matter and are known as 'anal-expulsives'. Fixations at the phallic stage may lead to a 'phallic' personality. Such persons are self-preoccupied, intrusive, noisy, inconsiderate, and self-aggrandizing.

Freud meant much more by sexuality than a mere impulse toward sexual union. He used the word sex rather broadly and attributed a sexual component to a variety of emotions. Sympathy, affiliation, loyalty, friendship, filial devotion, parental affection, piety, romantic love and even aesthetic feelings were all considered to be sublimated forms of sexual attachments.

THE TECHNIQUE OF PSYCHOANALYSIS

The psychoanalysis is based upon the premise that human behaviour is determined largely by unconscious psychological forces. Therefore, the general goal of the therapy is to make the client aware of the unconscious, psychological forces that are causing him or her difficulty, and to bring about a fundamental change in the client's personality so that he is released from his neurotic disorders. Freud believed that neurosis was caused by the repression of disturbing feelings and emotions associated with conflicts established in early childhood. These conflicts result from the impulses of the id and/or the strictures of an overdemanding superego. He assumed that the patient's ego was too weak to cope with such conflicts and defended itself by repressing them into the unconscious. However, conflicts do not go away; they find expression through the symptoms and neurotic behaviour of the client. Once unconscious motives or needs are acknowledged, they can presumably be dealt with in a more realistic and adaptive way.

However, the client must not only achieve insight into the cause of his or her symptoms but must also experience the emotion associated with the original memory. Before therapy the client's ego defends itself by repressing the conflict into the unconscious; after therapy, the client's ego is stronger and capable of handling the demands of the id, superego and external reality in a more mature manner. Thus, psychoanalytic therapy can be considered to comprise two stages:

(1) the release of repression, thereby allowing the conflict to enter consciousness, and

(2) the re-direction of the emotional energy (libido) associated with the repression, thereby allowing the client's ego to gain control of the conflict.

The analyst achieves this end in three ways. (1) by encouraging the client to build up an emotional relationship, or transference with the analyst, (2) by getting the client to freely associate about past thoughts and experiences – by interpreting these free associations, the analyst can often discover both the content and the dynamics of the client's unconscious mental processes – and (3) by the analysis of the symbolization of dreams reported by the client.

Free association

Freud developed the technique of free association in his attempts to dredge up all the unconscious drives and repressions that were, in his view, the fount of neurotic behaviour. He had tried hypnosis as a means of lowering conscious defences to such horrendous self-knowledge, but he was not a skilled hypnotist nor was every client susceptible to hypnotism. He therefore devised a technique which would effectively enable him to delve into the unconscious levels of the human psyche. That technique was free association and it is often termed the 'basic rule' for without it no psychoanalytic therapy can proceed.

Free association is the process whereby the client is told to tell the therapist without censorship whatever thought, feeling, or memory enters his or her mind. Considerations of shame, impropriety, triviality and so on are to be abandoned, and absolutely anything that comes into one's mind is to be related. In one of his few papers on technique (1913), Freud wrote that he would say the following to a patient:

> So say whatever goes through your mind. Act as though, for instance, you were a traveller sitting next to the window of a railway carriage and describing to someone inside the carriage the changing views which you see outside. Finally, never forget that you have promised to be absolutely honest, and never leave anything out because, for some reason or other, it is unpleasant to tell it (p. 135).

So the client is encouraged to say anything that comes to mind, no matter how silly, illogical or painful the thought may seem. If one thought triggers other thoughts or images, the client should report them all. Psychoanalysts believe that free association is the main tool for revealing the contents of the unconscious mind. But Freud did not view free association as simply random utterances. He maintained that, like all mental events, the thought processes governing it are determined.

At first the client's utterances are awkward and guarded. This is because the 'basic rule' of free association – to say everything that comes to mind, without selection, without editing – is a very difficult one to follow. The client has spent a lifetime learning self-control, learning to be cautious and to think before speaking. The open expression of sexual and aggressive feelings is generally thought unacceptable for children and adults in our society, we are taught to inhibit or repress these feelings. Yet sexual and aggressive feelings are a main focus in psychoanalysis, since they are the major drives of the id.

Even an individual who tries conscientiously to follow the rule will fail to tell many things. Some passing thoughts seem to be too important to mention, some too stupid others too indiscreet.

Suppose for example, that a woman's freedom is being hampered because she must care for her invalid mother. Under such circumstances, she may unconsciously wish for the relief that her mother's death might bring. But she would disapprove of such a death wish because it would be a violation of love and loyalty. Actually, this death wish may be very near to awareness, but the habits of a lifetime make the woman deny it even to herself. She may show a preoccupation with death in her fantasies or in other ways: possibly she hums tunes that are played at funerals. By acknowledging these fleeting thoughts instead of repressing them, she becomes aware of previously unrecognized ideas and feelings that are close to awareness. With practice, she gradually brings to consciousness ideas and feelings that have been deeply repressed.

People unconsciously repress or resist the recall of certain thoughts and feelings because they fear that to acknowledge them will be threatening or degrading. The therapist aids them in overcoming this resistance. Sometimes a person has a free flow of associations until something blocks the way. Then the mind seems to go blank, and the client can think of nothing to say. This blankness presumably represents resistance to the recall of something effectively repressed. Sometimes after a particularly revealing session, the client may forget the next appointment – another indication of resistance to disclosing what is hidden. But as an atmosphere of trust develops, the client becomes more comfortable and more skilful at free association, particularly as whatever he reports is neither condemned nor condoned, simply listened to by the therapist.

Transference

In psychoanalysis, the client's attitudes toward the analyst are considered important in determining progress. Sooner or later the client develops strong emotional responses to the psychoanalyst, perhaps admiring him or her greatly in one session but showing scorn in the next. This tendency to make the therapist the object of emotional response is known as transference. Freud first noticed transference when he realized that clients ascribed to him characteristics of God and the devil or professed mad love for him even though their meetings were brief and infrequent. Many modern analysts believe that the handling of the transference is the key to successful analysis. By becoming a father figure, the analyst encourages the client to react towards him as he did (perhaps inappropriately) toward significant figures in his childhood.

In transference the client comes to perceive the therapist as an especially important person. The client may become very demanding of the therapist, or very dependent, behaving like a child toward its parent. According to the theory, by experiencing these childlike thoughts and feelings toward the therapist or father figure the client is in a position to gain true insight into previously unconscious thoughts and feelings about others, usually parents. To cite one example: A young woman being treated by a woman psychoanalyst remarked one day as she entered the analyst's office, 'I'm glad you're not wearing those lace collars you wore the last several times I was here. I don't like them on you'. During the hour, the analyst pointed out that she had not in fact worn any lace collars. During the preceding sessions, the client had assigned to the analyst the role of the client's mother, and had falsely pictured the analyst as dressing as her mother had dressed when the client was a child and was undergoing the emotionally disturbing experiences being discussed with the analyst. The client, while surprised, accepted the interpretation and thereby gained understanding of transference.

Transference does not always involve false perceptions; often the client simply expresses feelings toward the analyst that he or she had felt toward figures who were important earlier in life. On the basis of these expressed feelings, the analyst is able to interpret the nature of the displaced impulses. For example, a man who has always admired an older brother detects something in the analyst's attitude that reminds him of the brother. An angry attack on the analyst may lead to the uncovering of hostile feelings toward his brother that the person had never acknowledged before.

As the client relives these emotionally charged past experiences, the therapist provides tolerant and understanding support. The therapist helps the client see how these reactions express past conflicts, and how they disrupt the client's present life. At this stage of therapy, the transference relationship with the therapist can be replaced by a more mature and realistic relationship. Then the client can begin to approach his or her life problems in a rational and effective manner.

The transference process is crucial to therapy, for without it the analyst's interpretations would never even be considered by the client. In fact, Freud argues that psychoanalytic therapy has little effect on clients suffering from certain types of mental illness, such as depression, paranoia and schizophrenia, because such persons are unable to produce transference. According to Freud, these diseases originate from repressed conflicts, but for some reason reduce the client's capacity for transference. The clients remain totally indifferent to the analyst and can therefore not be influenced by him.

Dream analysis

In his book *The Interpretation of Dreams*, Freud (1900) maintained that it was useful to consider dreams as representing, in a symbolic way, the unconscious conflicts or desires of the dreamer. When a person is asleep, since defences are lowered, repressed, unconscious material can emerge through the symbolism of dreams. The disturbing material which is striving to gain expression through a dream is referred to as the latent content of the dream. It is this content to which the analyst is trying to gain access. The description of the dream as reported is called the manifest content of the dream. The latent content is transformed into the manifest content of the dream by a number of unconscious distorting processes which Freud referred to collectively as dream work. He regarded the dream as the 'royal road to the unconscious'. The purpose of the symbolic nature of the dream message is to avoid anxiety that would wake the person up. The symbolic meaning of elements of a dream cannot easily be interpreted without knowing the associational links of the individual who had the dream. Freud believed that sexual conflicts determined most symbols. Although Freud proposed that such general symbolism may be involved, he felt that each person tends to have idiosyncratic associations that lead to unique symbols as well. It is the therapist's task to discover the meaning of such symbols.

After the client has related a dream, the analyst asks the person to free associate to various elements of the dream. He may also ask for information about the previous day in an effort to understand the manifest content (the superficial story of the dream), and the latent content (the symbolic meaning of that story). For example, a woman reported dreaming that a man unknown to her stole her car and was killed in an accident – the manifest content. The latent content of her dream was not obvious and could be clarified only with free association and the therapist's knowledge of some of the personality dynamics of the client. However, the latent content became clear when the therapist discovered that the unknown man could be considered a symbol for her husband.

The woman did not know or understand her husband very well ('unknown to her'), he frequently took advantage of her ('stole her car'), and she was very angry at him for this manipulative behaviour ('he was killed'). Her anger toward him was unacceptable to her, and she feared expressing it because she felt he would leave her. The anxiety-provoking latent content of the dream was expressed symbolically.

Although Freud acknowledged that the interpretation of dream symbols was incomplete, he nonetheless described the analysis of symbolism as the most remarkable part of his dream theory. The basis for this evaluation was his conviction that symbolism is a general property of unconscious thought and by no means confined to dreams. Freud assumed that virtually every social act has an unconscious and, therefore, symbolic component that may be analysed and interpreted.

According to Freud, a number of symbolized objects can be placed in three categories. The first refers to parents and siblings; parents are represented by royalty: kings, queens, emperors, chiefs, presidents, lords and ladies; children, brothers and sisters appear as rats, mice, squirrels, frogs, and foxes.

The second category, by far the largest, contains sexual symbols. The male sexual organ is represented by: sticks, umbrellas, poles, trees, knives, daggers, pistols, taps, pencils, reptiles, fish. The female sexual anatomy is represented by: pits, caves, jars, bottles, cupboards, doors and gates. Losing teeth symbolizes castration, while blossoms and flowers represent virginity.

The third category contains symbols of a broader and more Jungian variety. Birth is symbolized by going into or coming out of water, a symbol presumably derived from man's evolutionary origins as an aquatic animal and from the liquid environment of the amniotic sac.

Symptomatic acts

Another route into the unconscious is via the errors and mistakes of everyday life, so-called Freudian slips. In his book *The Psychopathology of Everyday Life* (1901), Freud suggested that repressed material can find expression through behaviour which is beyond conscious control, slips of the tongue, changes in behaviour toward the therapy hour, forgetting therapy appointments, and unusual behaviour during therapy may all be symptomatic of deeper and more significant unconscious processes.

Resistance

Freud recognized a perplexing fact from the beginning of his psychoanalytic treatment of clients. Although clients willingly came for treatment because they were suffering, and although there was only one fundamental rule of the treatment, free association, clients continually 'broke' this rule. They censored thoughts, feelings, and memories; sometimes they did not want to talk, and sometimes nothing came to the patient's mind although he or she was trying to associate. Clients wanted to be helped but, paradoxically, they would not consistently free associate, the one necessary input into the treatment from the clients that would allow Freud to help them. This behaviour, termed resistance, is hypothesized to have many motivations. Clients resist primarily because they feel anxious, and anxiety was the reason that a thought or feeling was originally repressed. In treatment these same 'unacceptable' thoughts and so on still make clients anxious, and they do not want to allow these thoughts to be conscious or to allow the therapist to be aware of such thoughts. Thus clients 'hold back', even though expressing the thoughts is necessary to the treatment. Like transference, resistance is ubiquitous. Resistance is both normal and the main hindrance to alleviating the client's distress. Indeed, a major goal of dynamic treatment is systematically to help the client gain insight into the particular resistances used. Resistance interferes with the ultimate success of the treatment only if it is unanalysable. The client is helped to comprehend how he misperceives and misunderstands his own experience by gaining insight into his defence processes and resistance.

Interpretation

The psychoanalyst's basic job is interpretation, explaining to the client the unconscious meaning of what he or she says. The purpose of interpretation is to help the client overcome the resistance to remembering repressed memories. Not infrequently the symbolic meaning of what is being said is not obvious, and the analyst must maintain a free-floating attention for many sessions, looking for clues to the content of the unconscious mind.

Once he develops a degree of certainty about his interpretation, the analyst must decide when to present it to the client. If the interpretation is given before the client is capable of accepting it, anxiety will be generated and the repression will become more severe. It is desirable to lead clients slowly so that they can gradually arrive at their own interpretations and work at overcoming their own resistance.

A single proper interpretation does not resolve the client's problems. The repression of unconscious material shows up in various aspects of the person's life, and repeated interpretations are required to help the person give up the repression in all aspects of his or her life. The process of repeated interpretation and continued efforts on the part of the client to resolve the conflict is called working through.

Abreaction, insight and working through

The course of improvement during psychoanalytic therapy is commonly attributed to three main experiences: abreaction, gradual insight into one's difficulties, and the repeated working through of conflicts and one's reactions to them. A person experiences abreaction when he or she freely expresses a repressed emotion or relives an intense emotional experience. The process is also called 'catharsis', as though it were a kind of emotional cleansing. Such free expression may bring some relief but by itself does not eliminate the causes of conflict. In psychoanalytic therapy, abreaction (or catharsis) is accompanied by interpretations that help the individual understand the conflicts revealed. Thus, the benefits from catharsis under these circumstances do not contradict experimental results, which report that expressing aggression fails to reduce subsequent aggressive responses.

A person achieves insight when he or she understands the roots of the conflict. Sometimes insight comes when the client recovers the memory of a repressed experience, but the popular notion that a psychoanalytic cure typically results from the sudden recall of a single dramatic episode is mistaken. The individual's troubles seldom have a single source, and insight comes through a gradual increase in self-knowledge. Insight and abreaction must work together; clients must understand their feelings and feel what they understand. The reorientation is never simply intellectual.

As analysis progresses, the client goes through a lengthy process of re-education known as working through. By examining the same conflicts over and over again as they have appeared in a variety of situations, the person learns to face, rather than to deny, reality and to react in more mature and effective ways. By working through these conflicts during therapy, the person becomes strong enough to face the threat of the original conflict situation and to react to it without undue anxiety.

The end result claimed for a successful psychoanalysis is a deep-seated modification of the personality that makes it possible for the individual to cope with problems on a realistic basis, without the recurrence of the problems that brought him or her to treatment.

Psychoanalysis typically takes from 2–5 years to complete, and the 50 minute-long therapy sessions are usually held 3–5 times a week. The most successful clients seem to be between 15 and 50 years of age. They must be bright, verbal, self-motivated, and willing to co-operate with the therapist. Although psychoanalysis is occasionally used with individuals classed as 'psychotic', the usual client is a mildly disturbed or neurotic individual.

There are no set rules governing when dynamic therapy terminates. Analysis is generally not considered complete until the transference neurosis is cured. Ideally, dynamic therapies end when the working through is complete. What this tautology means is dependent upon the goals of the client, the goals of the therapist, the theoretical orientation of the therapist, and the fact that, as Freud pointed out (1937, 216–253), analysis (or therapy) is interminable. What Freud meant by this is that because conflict is always a product of civilization, and defence always accompanies conflict, it is impossible for the therapy to be completely over. Most basically put, therapy ends optimally when a client has insight into the core difficulties that interfered with his loving and working, and when he has integrated this insight fully enough into his character to then have the choice about whether or not he wishes to change.

EVALUATION

In the 80 year history of psychoanalytic practice surprisingly little has been learnt about its therapeutic value. Excluding single case-reports, retrospective surveys and non-controlled clinical reports, there are only four studies in which any form of research control was introduced, and the conclusions that can be drawn from these few sources are limited or unsatisfactory or both.

(Rachman and Wilson, 1980, p. 50)

This is how one major British text sums up psychoanalysis. This is mainly because an evaluation of psychoanalysis presents numerous difficulties. The most serious of these is how to deal with the bias that operates in the selection of clients, and the related problem of premature terminations of treatment. The very high rate of premature terminations of treatment suggests a serious deficiency in the criteria and techniques used by psychoanalysts in selecting clients for treatment.

Psychoanalytic theory has its own and quite distinctive diagnostic concepts, criteria of success, definition of the nature of a failure, and perhaps central to all these, the purpose of treatment. For example, Grünbaum (1977) quotes the claims of Erich Fromm: 'Many patients have experienced a new sense of vitality and capacity for joy, and no other method than psychoanalysis could have produced these changes'. Most often, it is claimed that the purpose of psychoanalysis is to improve the total functioning of the client's personality. Unfortunately, the claims are as extravagant as they are vague. How, for example, a 'sense of vitality' or a 'capacity for joy' can be assessed reliably and validly is never made clear, nor does it seem possible to do so.

The most important criticisms brought to bear against psychoanalysis are considered below.

Therapy forces the client into a preconceived theoretical structure. If the client disagrees with the analyst's explanation of his problem he may discontinue therapy, in which case an analyst regards him as showing resistance, rather than the therapy as inappropriate.

Therapy incorporates a value system. For example, it is considered perverse for an individual to be dependent, homosexual or a perfectionist. Clients undergoing Freudian psychoanalysis are in effect moulded into people who would have been acceptable to the Viennese middle class of 60 or 70 years ago.

Therapy is limited in terms of the types of clients for which it is suitable – it has been found that the type of people accepted for treatment tend to be young, attractive, verbal, intelligent and successful (the YAVIS effect). This is true for all types of psychotherapy. Most analysts would admit that, because of the emphasis placed on accurate verbal communication in psychoanalysis, it is necessary for clients to be of a reasonable intellectual level. It has also been found that middle class clients tend to receive psychoanalysis, whereas working class clients tend to be assigned to a behaviour therapist. Freud's theories were based on his experiences with a small and atypical sample of people, generally wealthy, middle-class neurotic Viennese Jewish women, some of whom had been attracted to Freud because of the sort of explanations and treatment that he offered, and who served to fan the flames of his ideas by accepting his interpretations and analysis.

The therapeutic effectiveness of analysis has never been shown to be particularly significant. Eysenck (1952) has claimed that of those persons receiving psychotherapy, 67 per cent show an improvement after treatment. However, he also found that the same percentage exhibit 'spontaneous remission', that is, recover with no treatment at all. This suggests that psychotherapy has little or no effect. However, because the technical problems involved in such assessment are so immense (for instance, researchers have difficulty agreeing on what counts as a cure), it can only be concluded that the validity of psychodynamic theory as a therapeutic method has not yet been proved. Moreover, Fiedler (1950) showed that the amount of therapist's experience is a greater determinant of psychotherapeutic outcome than whether he/she is a Freudian, Jungian or whatever.

Many of the concepts of psychodynamic theory are rather loosely defined, or defined only by reference to other concepts within the theory. This means that it is difficult, if not impossible, to define these concepts in terms of observable behaviour in any precise fashion. As a corollary they cannot be tested in any experiment. There are many metaphors and analogies which can, but need not, be taken literally. Examples would be latency, death instinct, Oedipus complex and castration anxiety. Does castration anxiety refer to the fear of loss of the penis, or does it refer to the child's fear of injury to his body, at a time that his body image is of increased importance to his self esteem?

Psychodynamic theory contains a number of ideas which, by their all-encompassing nature, enable a psychodynamic explanation to be given for every possible action. For example, in psychoanalytic theory, fixation at the anal stage of psychosexual development can lead either to stinginess or excessive generosity in the individual's behaviour. The concept of 'reaction formation' for example, enables the psychoanalyst to explain contrasting and contradictory behaviour as resulting from the same mechanisms. The theory is thus able to explain everything after the event, but is very weak at predicting what will happen, and the ability to predict is an important feature of a scientific theory.

That the psychodynamic approach contains elements which lead to contrary predictions must weaken its claim to be regarded as scientific. For any body of theory to be accepted as a valid scientific perspective, its consequences must be statable as hypotheses which are capable of being refuted through empirical investigation. The hypothesis that fixation at the anal stage can lead either to stinginess or to the opposite, generosity, is evidently not refutable; whatever the outcome, the theory can account for it. To that extent the psychodynamic approach fails to meet the criteria of a scientific theory. But it may be that we are trying to judge Freudian theory with an inappropriate 'paradigm', in that a theory is held to be scientific if it is capable of being falsified, that is, if it can be put to some crucial test which might prove it wrong. But Freudian theory undertakes to explain completely opposing facts: if a client loves his mother, it is because of his Oedipus complex: if he hates her, it is reaction-formation to his Oedipus complex: if he is indifferent to her, he has repressed his Oedipal feelings. In addition, there is the strong possibility that the psychoanalyst will put words into the mouths of his clients and interpret what they say in the light of the theory, thus finding what he expected.

The conventional experimental paradigm we use would claim that the data on which Freud built up his theories were not sound. The free associations of his clients and the recollections of their dreams, though interesting and thought provoking are not a sufficient base on which to erect a grand theory. They do not measure up to the standards of scientific data – they cannot be quantified, their reliability cannot be checked, memory may be subjective and selective and there is no use of control groups. In addition to these rather weighty reservations there is a sort of Freudian 'Catch 22', for Freud demanded that one had to believe in psychoanalysis before one was in a position to criticize it. This suggests faith rather than proof is the criterion.

Moreover, Freud was not really concerned with experimental verification. He wrote to one American researcher:

'I have examined your experimental studies for the verification of psychoanalytic assertions with interest. I cannot put much value on these confirmations because the wealth of reliable observations on which these assertions rest make them independent of experimental verification. Still, it (experimental verification) can do no harm.' (Quoted by Mackinnon and Dukes, 1962, p. 763)

His 'deterministic' theory is not well received by those such as the phenomenologists who regard man as having choice in his selection of behaviour (Chapter 12).

It could be argued that he held an unwholesome over-pessimistic and negative view of the human condition; that unhappiness is inescapable so that the most we can achieve even with therapeutic intervention is the mastery of some of the sources of our misery. Psychological health is in the psychoanalytical creed an ideal not a statistical norm.

But from a practical standpoint, psychoanalytic therapy has the disadvantage for clients that it involves a great deal of expense, in terms of both time and money. Further, during the course of analysis the client may be psychologically vulnerable and helpless for a long period. This is because at one stage in analysis the client's old defences and resistances have been broken down, yet the patient's ego is still not strong enough to cope adequately with the conflict. To overcome these problems, many analysts, who base their work on Freudian principles, carry out what is called psychoanalytically oriented psychotherapy. This is an abbreviated form of Freudian psychoanalysis, in which the analyst plays a much more directive role in manipulating the transference and in determining those areas which are thought to be significant to the client's neurosis. This type of psychotherapy employs psychoanalytic psychology to formulate and understand the client's difficulty and as a basis for treatment technique. It is a less intense form of therapy than psychoanalysis; clients are usually seen less frequently and need not necessarily free associate. At present, psychoanalytic clinicians in the United States and Britain are experimenting with extremely brief (e.g. 12–20 session) forms of therapy that focus intensively on the client's core or nuclear conflict. These clinicians claim that the new, brief, analytic therapies are highly effective. Psychoanalytic psychotherapy has become increasingly popular, even among those trained to practice psychoanalysis, and today considerably more clients are treated with psychoanalytic psychotherapy than with psychoanalysis.

But despite this major effort to widen the scope of psychoanalysis, by and large the treatment remains most clearly suited for neurotic problems, in contrast to psychoses or other kinds of severe impairments, such as alcoholism, where the person's life is, practically speaking, out of control. It is also not designed for situations where an acute problem is closely associated with a sudden environmental change. It is most indicated when the neurotic problems – which may include sexual difficulties, disturbances in mood and general impairment of personal relations, as well as the more classical symptoms – are diffuse and relatively chronic, and when they are felt subjectively. In other words, the neurosis should be experienced mainly as something within oneself, not simply between oneself and the rest of the world.

On the credit side, Freud made major contributions to psychology and greatly influenced the developmental approach. Psychoanalysis has led to the utilization of new techniques, such as those of free association and dream interpretation, and has been a significant force in the development and utilization of projective techniques in the assessment of personality.

Freud transformed man's view of man as well as introducing such areas as 'the unconscious', 'dreams', 'repression' as worthy of consideration in any attempt to understand human behaviour. His presentation of 'normal' life as differing only in degree from neurotic behaviour was salutory.

Psychoanalysis, the new technique that he discovered, was the first dynamic psychotherapy, and it is the foundation for all future ones. Freud's theory and technique revolutionized the understanding and treatment of mental disorders.

As an observer of human behaviour, and as a person with a creative imagination, Freud was indeed a genius with few, if any, equals. The theory he developed certainly has the virtue of being comprehensive. The richness of his observations and the attention he paid to all details of human behaviour, was such that few other therapies give comparable attention to the functioning of the individual as a whole.

It is possible to restate the theories in a way which is scientifically testable. Thus psychoanalytic theory, as a whole, can be broken down into a series of testable hypotheses, for it is not a unitary theory but, rather a collection of theories. Objective research can then be carried out into these hypotheses. Kline (1972) has made a significant contribution in gathering together, in an evaluative survey, a large number of research papers that purport to study Freudian concepts, such as anal and oral characters, castration anxiety, etc. He is by no means uncritical and his careful discussion of the evidence shows him to be concerned with the niceties of scientific proof to a degree which is distinctly missing in many Freudians. His conclusion is that 'any blanket rejection of Freudian theory as a whole (e.g. Eysenck, 1952) simply flies in the face of the evidence'.

Whether we agree or disagree with Freudian thought we must acknowledge that Freud has influenced the ideas and methods of psychiatry and clinical psychology far more than any other person. Freud's impact is also clear in other disciplines including anthropology, history, literature and the arts. In short, Freud's thinking has had a monumental influence on our culture.

Further reading

Appignanesi, R. and Zarate, O. (1979). *Freud for Beginners*. (London: Readers and Writers' Publishing Co-op)
Brown, J. A. C. (1961). *Freud and the Post-Freudians*. (Harmondsworth: Penguin)
Jones, E. (1964). *The Life and Work of Sigmund Freud*. (Harmondsworth: Penguin)
Kline, P. (1972). *Fact and Fantasy in Freudian Theory*. (London: Methuen)

Chapter 3

NEO-FREUDIAN APPROACHES

Although neo-Freudians form a diverse group they tend to possess in common some central themes which are quite dissonant from Freudian tenets of faith. They generally reject Freud's theory of libido since for them sexuality is considered a result of character rather than the cause of character. In neo-Freudian psychotherapy emphasis is placed on a person's interpersonal relationships and their relationship to society; with as a corollary an emphasis on aspects of mental activity that reflect the interpersonal world such as self evaluation, striving, assertiveness, security and acceptance by others. So they consider libido and instinct theories to be outdated; the individual's adaptation to his or her environment is the crucial behavioural variable. Concepts such as the Oedipus complex, formation of the superego, anxiety and inferiority feelings are seen as products of our culture. They all believe that biology determines behaviour less than culture, which is seen as quite malleable. The neo-Freudians tend to be more optimistic than Freud; as persons can perfect society, so can they perfect themselves.

There are, of course, areas of continuity with Freudian thought, in particular an emphasis on development and childhood experience. Neuroses are still seen as unassimilated particles of infantile life, and analysis – i.e. resolving current experience into its neurotic elements through verbal exploration – is still the major means of intervention. Nonetheless, there is a shift of focus and of emphasis out of which emerges a positive human image distinctly different from Freud's negative version, an ego driven organism rather than an id dominated one.

The early neo-Freudians, Adler and Jung, were rebels who felt that Freud was essentially wrong but later neo-Freudians still associate themselves with Freud while at the same time attempting to correct Freud's lack of emphasis on socio-cultural and interpersonal factors. Few neo-Freudians apart from Adler and Jung have produced therapeutic applications of their theories.

JUNG'S ANALYTIC PSYCHOLOGY

THEORY

Jung was one of Freud's most promising students who broke with the psychoanalytic school over its emphasis on sexuality, and developed his own theory and therapeutic method known as analytical psychology. Jung still accepted the basic concepts of psychodynamics as put forward by Freud, but created his own theories of the psyche and personality. Jung introduced many new concepts, e.g. extrovert, introvert and complex, as well as devising the word-association test. Jung never fully accepted the theory of infantile sexuality that Freud considered the touchstone of psychoanalysis.

In the Jungian model, behaviour is still driven by the libido, but Jung's libido is non-sexual and represents the life force which underlies all natural phenomena, including the human psyche. For Jung, the libido is life itself and sexuality is only one manifestation of it. Similarly, Jung accepts Freud's notion of psychosexual development as a series of stages related to bodily functions, but he redefines the stages and associated conflicts, such as the Oedipus complex, in terms of his own idea of psychodynamics.

The psyche

In speaking of the mind and mental activity, Jung uses the terms *psyche* and *psychic* – which cover both the conscious and the unconscious. The psyche is composed of three levels in fact:

> Consciousness
> Personal unconscious and
> Collective unconscious.

Jung's conception of the psyche is of a system which is dynamic, in constant movement and at the same time, self regulating. Libido is the motive force in Jung's psychology. It flows between two opposing poles,

PROGRESSION	←——→	REGRESSION
CONSCIOUSNESS	←——→	UNCONCIOUSNESS
EXTROVERSION	←——→	INTROVERSION
THINKING	←——→	FEELING

These opposites have a regulating function; when one extreme is reached, libido passes over into the opposite. e.g. violent rage succeeded by calm.

This regulating function is, to Jung, inherent in human nature, with the natural movement of the libido being forward and backward.

FORWARD   - SATISFIES CONSCIOUS DEMANDS   - PROGRESSION
BACKWARD - SATISFIES UNCONSCIOUS   - REGRESSION.
                    DEMANDS

Regression is a normal counterpole to progression. This is not necessarily bad and can be looked upon as a restorative phase, a strategic retreat. Normal regression is a necessity of life. By performing regression, the ego may discover useful knowledge in the unconscious that will enable the person to overcome a present obstacle.

The conscious mind or ego is made up of conscious perceptions, memories, thoughts and feelings. It is responsible for the individual's feeling of identity. The personal unconscious corresponds to Freud's concept of the unconscious, with the addition that it contains personal experiences which have been discarded as they are no longer pertinent to the life of the individual. However, the personal unconscious is only a small fraction of the unconscious, the vast bulk of which is known as the collective unconscious, as it contains the collective beliefs and myths of the race to which the individual belongs. The collective unconscious itself can be divided into sub-levels. As you go deeper into the collective unconscious it becomes more universal. The knowledge stored there is considered as common to all humanity, the psychological heritage of humanities and deeper still the knowledge relates to man's primate and animal ancestry.

A common visual analogy used to illustrate Jung's concept of the psyche is shown in Figure 2. In this figure the parts of the islands above water represent the conscious minds of different individuals; the part of the island below the water is the personal unconscious; deeper still is the rock on which groups of islands stand and this represents the radical/collective unconscious (e.g. Negroid, Aryan, Mongolian groups, etc.). The sea bed on which all the islands ultimately stand corresponds to the universal collective unconscious which contains the psychological heritage of humanity as a whole, even relating back to its primate ancestry. In Jung's words, 'The collective unconscious contains the whole spiritual heritage of mankind's evolution born anew in the brain structure of every individual' (Jung, 1960, p. 158), as a whole of animal life and of man's primate ancestors. It is the psychic residue of man's evolutionary development, a residue of repeated experiences over many generations. It is almost entirely detached from anything personal in the life of an individual and it is seemingly universal. This area exercises a guiding influence over what a person learns as a result of experiences (e.g. latent fears strengthened by specific experiences in modern man). The collective unconscious has an important role in the Jungian system of psychotherapy. This is because it contains fundamental knowledge of humanity which is denied to consciousness. Jung attributed conflicts to a disturbance in the harmony of the total psyche – in other words, to an imbalance between the conscious and unconscious personal and collective factors which constitute the complex psyche. It is the collective unconscious which holds the key to the patient's problems, and it is by bringing the patient into contact with this level of the psyche that the therapist attempts to create a new equilibrium in the patient's psyche.

Jung based his notion of the collective unconscious on three types of observation:

(1) He noticed that the mythologies of widely different cultures contained very similar themes, e.g. the good but small person beats the bad big one as in Jack and the Beanstalk or David and Goliath.

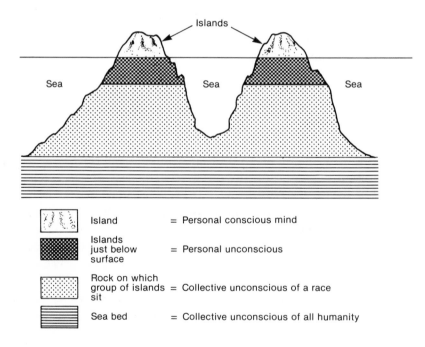

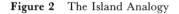
Figure 2   The Island Analogy

(2) The ideas found in mythology are also found time and again in the content of the fantasies of schizophrenics patients.

(3) In therapy Jung observed that the personal symbols which recur in clients' dreams bore little relation to their personal experience and gradually converge, over the course of analysis, toward the types of universal symbols employed in myths and legends. Typical examples of such universal symbols are the mother image, the child, sun-gods, the symbols of birth and rebirth.

The types of symbols referred to in (3) have an important role in Jung's model. Jung extended the Freudian concept of unconscious symbols, and thought of symbols as representing important aspects of living, usually in the form of concrete images. These images are personalized and appear in dreams, visions, fantasies and even art. Symbols are used by individuals to capture a multitude of feelings and ideas which are impossible to express in any other form.

The personal symbols employed by an individual have their origin in the personal unconscious. Universal symbols originate in the collective unconscious and transcend the differences between individuals. They relate to the common experience or knowledge of a race or species. These latter symbols are referred to as archetypes. There are a limited number of archetypal symbols corresponding to a relatively restricted range of situations basic to mankind as a whole.

Archetypes of the collective unconscious

Archetypes are the structural components of the collective unconscious. They were supposedly formed, during the thousands of years in which the human brain and human consciousness were emerging from an animal state. We become aware of them through certain typical images which recur in the psyche. An archetype is a universal thought form which contains large elements of emotion. It is a permanent deposit in the mind, of an experience that has constantly been repeated for many generations. This thought form creates images that correspond in normal waking life to some aspect of the conscious situation. Although all archetypes may be thought of as autonomous systems, relatively independent of the rest of the personality, some have evolved so far as to warrant their being treated as separate systems from the personality. These are:

The Persona, the Shadow, the Anima, the Animus and the Self

Persona

The persona is a mask behind which most people live. The individual must conform to the accepted norms of his society, and so he must repress disagreeable or inferior tendencies. This leads to a compromise between the individual and society as to what he should appear to be. The purpose of the mask is to make a definite impression on others, and may conceal the real nature of the individual. Society expects a role to be played reliably and consistently. Human nature is not consistent, yet in filling a role it must appear so. It is therefore inevitably falsified. It simplifies contacts by indicating what we may expect from others. Those who neglect the development of a persona, tend to offend others and have difficulty in establishing themselves in the world. However, there is danger in playing a role too well, as the individual becomes a mere reflection of society and completely denies the rest of his personality. The experiences from which this archetype develops consist of social interactions in which the assumption of a social role has served a useful purpose of man throughout his history as a social animal.

Shadow

The shadow archetype consists of primitive animal instincts which man inherited in his evolution from lower forms of life. It is the primitive, un-controlled part of ourselves. It is responsible for the conscious behaviour of unpleasant and socially reprehensible thoughts, feelings and actions. Thus the more restrictive the society in which we live, the larger will be our shadow. Such instincts may be hidden from public view by means of the persona, or repressed into the personal unconscious. The shadow is unavoidable and gives a three dimensional quality to the personality. Man is incomplete without it.

Anima and animus

Feminine and masculine traits occur in both sexes. Jung ascribes the feminine side of man's personality and the masculine side of woman's personality to archetypes. The feminine archetype in man is called the anima, the masculine archetype in woman is called the animus, and are the products of experience of man with woman. These archetypes cause each sex to manifest characteristics of the opposite sex and act as images which motivate each sex to respond and to understand the opposite sex.

Through contact with the opposite sex, the image becomes tangible. The first and most significant of these contacts is of the boy with his mother and of the girl with her father. The picture is formed and coloured by this encounter and by the innate capacity to produce an image of woman (anima) and man (animus). Later the image is projected on to the various encounters with the opposite sex. However, if these archetypal images are projected without any real regard for the character of the individual, discord may occur when it becomes apparent that there are discrepancies between the real and the ideal.

Both the anima and the animus are mediators between the conscious and the unconscious mind, and when they become personified in fantasies or dreams they present an opportunity to understand something that has hitherto been unconscious. Jung takes dreams seriously and considers them to be 'the voice of nature'. Understanding the significance of dreams and the influence of the unconscious, is a gain for the personality.

Two other archetypes considered by Jung are the *Old Wise Man* and the *Great Mother*. The former often represents the king, hero, saviour, etc. This can be a danger when awakened in man, as he may believe he possesses the wisdom and power that the archetype holds, compelling the man to act beyond his physical capacity. The parallel archetype is the Great Mother, which can be equally destructive.

Self

This represents man's striving for unity. It is the function which unites all opposing elements and in so doing transmutes them. The self is the mid-point of the personality. This archetype motivates man's behaviour, causing him to search for wholeness especially through the means of religion. Jung discovered this concept whilst observing oriental religions. The archetype of the self does not become evident until middle age, when the components of personality are fully developed.

THE PROCESS OF JUNGIAN THERAPY

Jungian treatment resembles what can be called 'supportive psycho-therapy': The client and analyst sit face to face, practical advice is dispensed, a sort of folk wisdom reigns, and neurotic behaviour is handled on a matter-of-fact, conscious level. The general attitude conveyed is that one's neurosis is part of a much larger whole. By attaining philosophic calm and detachment, the client prepares the way for that encounter with the transcendent towards which the Jungian aims.

Jung's approach includes a great deal of work on unconscious material, dreams and other art forms, which communicate from the depths of the personality both to the client himself as well as to the therapist. This work is carried out *between* therapist and client. They meet and spend an hour at

a time talking together. The number of times a week varies with individuals; at the beginning perhaps two or three times a week, later perhaps
about once a week or possibly less; it may continue for some years. But
Jung was always ready to adapt to the need of an individual's life. He said
that the psychological work or treatment should feed into the existing life
of an individual, and he encouraged everyone to continue living and
working normally if he could. Jung made it quite clear to all his students
that the psychotherapeutic work was the mutual responsibility of both
therapist and client.

The analytic or psychotherapeutic process usually consists in the client
telling his life story and 'confessing' his part in it. Emotion is discharged
in doing this, and the individual is often much relieved in the early stages.
The 'confession' is followed by explanation and a mutual discussion of
the problems that have arisen. The present situation is reviewed in the
light of the early years. Dreams or other art forms are studied and used to
expose the conscious situation to the modification and compensatory
influence of the unconscious. Jung insists that the doctor can only look on
and try to understand the attempts at restitution and cure which nature
herself is making, and that between conscious and unconscious there
exists a compensatory relationship. The unconscious always tries to make
whole the conscious part of the psyche by adding to it the parts that are
missing, and so prevent a dangerous loss of balance.

Jung says that a dream that is not understood remains a mere
occurrence; understood it becomes a living experience. For Jung,
Freud's view of the dream as a distorted representation of a hidden wish
was erroneous. The dream was the most notable way the archetypes had
of making themselves known. Therefore, the dream itself, the manifest
dream, was sacrosanct.

Thus Jung deliberately prohibited free association. Instead he used the
technique of amplification, expanding the dream content in dramatic
terms within the dreamer's life (as by asking the patient to imagine his
way further into the dream scenario), and then situating the forms of the
dream within the world tradition of myth and symbol. In this way the
dream itself was revealed to be a higher form of cognition, guiding the
client to a superordinate knowledge rather than leading to what he had to
hide.

Jung regarded this technique as the way to bring a person into greater
and greater contact with the deep unconscious; and this contact itself
without any external practice or mediation with the personal unconscious, was considered the main healing principle. Thus, Jung's
approach to dreams sometimes resembled the work of a modern biblical

Joseph than the modern analyst.

Just having a dream is argued as therapeutic by Jung, and this applies to all creative expression in whatever art form which springs from hidden and unconscious levels of experience. So much more, however, can be derived from the 'occurrence' if attention is given to it afterwards and some understanding of it achieved. Jung was one of the pioneers of art therapy. He used the creative expression of his students and clients, painting, writing, sculpture, etc., in the same way as he used dreams. The ego became involved and related to that which was previously unconscious. By receiving the mysterious messages within the dream, painting, sculpture, poetry, dance, mime, music and drama, created by the clients or students, modification, re-education and development takes place. Thus the life of the individual can be adjusted, balanced or radically changed from within the psyche itself.

Neurosis is seen as a conflict between unequally developed parts of personality rather than a conflict between emotional drives and society. Neurosis arises when the individual is inadequately equipped to deal with the adjustments needed to live in society. Such an individual may regress but, for Jung, this regression to a more archaic stage might provide a creative adaptation, in that the individual is calling upon reserves in the collective unconscious which might help him to cope. If, however, no solution is found in the collective unconscious the subject will regress further and neurosis sets in.

Therefore, Jung (like Adler) is more concerned with future goals rather than past history (as is Freud). For Jung a neurosis has an aim as well as a cause both of which have to be understood since the aim is an attempt, perhaps vain and inadequate, at psychological healing. The problem of neurosis or health is then one of integration between different parts of the person and that which is transpersonal, transcendent. The goal of therapy was to mend those splits. Thus Jung focused, in a way that no other has done, on problems of the middle and later years of life. The prime objective was to allow a person to experience the split-off parts of himself, especially the archetypal emissaries of the collective unconscious and certain other psychological formations, which were, so to speak, contiguous with it, such as the anima, or split-off female quality in the male (animus for the woman) and the shadow, a negative or inferior self-image. The goal of Jungian therapy is the rapprochement of the self with that which is beyond the person, yet expressive through him. Jung called this goal individuation – roughly translated as the attainment of wisdom.

The individuation process

This involves the development of the personality in the direction of stable unity. The individuated person must become aware of and accept his unconscious, while remaining aware of his unique personality and his relationship or 'brotherhood' with all living things. The process aims at the end product the 'whole man', which necessitates forging a link between the conscious and the unconscious aspects of the psyche.

Jung extends this idea to the realms of religion. He considers that this experience could also be formulated as the finding of the God within. Jung's view is that man possesses a 'natural religious function' and his psychic health and stability depend on this. This function influences him as powerfully as the instincts of sexuality and aggression. Nowadays the energy used for religion and ritual observance can find expression in such things as political creeds, or the remorseless pursuit of knowledge. But no completely rational system can fill the deepest human need – to relate the inner and outer man in equal degree. Organized religion is a channel which controls the unruly influences of the collective unconscious. Man needs to experience the god-image within himself, and to feel it correspond to the forms that his religion gives to it. If this does not happen, there can be a split in his nature: he may be outwardly civilized, but inwardly barbarian. The individuation process can help the individual who finds in the 'Christian drama' no satisfactory expression of his needs.

Jungian therapy is for both neurotics and 'normal' middle-aged persons who find life empty and meaningless. Jung believed that adulthood was an important period of psychological growth and that spiritual development was vital to the healthy personality.

EVALUATION

Jung led a long, productive life but he did not exert as much influence on psychotherapy as might have been thought. Jung's impact may be seen in the work of Herman Rorschach, the founder of the projective inkblot test, and in the character typological work of psychologists such as Eysenck (although Eysenck's emphasis is quite different). The Jungians were and are primarily located in Switzerland and London. Today there is a renaissance of interest in Jung that accompanies a renewed interest in mysticism and Far-Eastern philosophy and religion. Jungian psychology is a creative scheme, however, that emphasizes very different aspects of human experience from Freudian psychology. It is a more optimistic view of human nature and potential.

Jungians claim that their method works well with every type of emotional disturbance, but that it is especially designed for the normal individual in middle life or beyond who seeks wisdom and enlightenment, but those to whom Jung's view of the universe does not represent truth would have to regard it as mystifying, since it replaces mundane and material explanations with transcendent ones.

In free-association analysis the client and the analyst produce associations during this co-operative procedure. Therefore, it is hardly surprising that the material or data produced is Jungian in content, since the analyst already has a pre-conceived idea of the collective unconscious. Jung's system can therefore be seen to be more indoctrinal than others.

Many analysts have argued against the necessity for a collective unconscious and its associated archetypes as psychic entities. They believe that it is only necessary to propose different strata of common knowledge and experience according to the degree of commonality between individuals in societies, cultures and even species. For them there is no clear dividing line between the material in the personal unconscious and that in the collective unconscious; both types of knowledge are learnt. For example, two people born and bred in Western society may have very different past histories, but will share the common experiences associated with education, which may not be true for a member of a primitive tribe in the Third World. However, all three individuals will have common experiences relating to human characteristics such as birth, death, parentage, dependence on sun and moon. Hence recurring symbols are hardly surprising. Jung's distinction between the collective and personal unconscious may therefore be rather arbitrary.

Jung had a wide knowledge of the religion, philosophy, myths and symbolism of many cultures, and he put this to use in his psychological studies. For this reason Jung has been criticized for being metaphysical rather than scientific in his theories. He does, however, have a great following – particularly amongst Catholic writers, e.g. Father Victor White. But on the whole, his work has had relatively less appeal or use for the psychologist or psychiatrist than other therapies covered in this book.

ADLERIAN PSYCHOTHERAPY

THE THEORY

Adler, originally a colleague of Freud, formed his own brand of psychotherapy, after he broke with Freud over the latter's insistence on the primacy of sexual instincts. Adler preferred a more social approach and substituted self-assertion as the prime motivating force. Alfred Adler called his psychology 'Individual Psychology', because he saw in a human being not a bundle of drives and instincts, but an indivisible unity, as in the meaning of the Latin word *individuum,* 'not to be broken into parts'.

Adler believed that the inferiority complex was the main cause of neurosis, and that every neurosis can be understood as an attempt to free oneself from a feeling of inferiority in order to gain a feeling of superiority. Neurosis enables symptoms to be used as an excuse, or to avoid situations or to gain control by emotional blackmail, e.g. presumed handicaps and psychosomatic illnesses. A common neurosis is one where a person has poor social relationships due to inferiority complex; he is bound up too much with his own prestige, is always on the defensive trying to prove himself and every contact is regarded as a rival. So neuroses develop from attempts to compensate for inferiority feelings. Such inferiority was seen by Adler to stem from the frustration of the main drive or motive he ascribed to man, that of self-assertion.

Adler's self-assertion is not Freud's aggression renamed. It is a need to be accepted by others, to achieve something, to be approved of. Self-assertion is liable to frustration in everyone at some time, but especially in childhood and in persons with mental or physical handicaps. 'To be a human being means to feel oneself inferior', wrote Adler. He believed that every human being requires security and that the small child with his intelligence far surpassing his physical power has a keen appreciation of his own inadequacy. A feeling of inferiority is created at birth as man is born into the world incomplete and unfulfilled. Everything that lies before the baby is better, bigger and more competent than he. As he grows his perceptive system makes him aware of his inferior role in society, and he is continuously reminded that most of the creatures around him can reach things, throw things, prepare things and control things much better than he can. Feeling inferior, he wishes to emulate the strengths and capacities of others. In a few abnormal cases, the child remains at an inferior level, is unable to try anything new, or reverts to an even more inferior role, but most humans want to go beyond where they are, as does the child who desires to be more complete than he is at any given moment in his early development. Once having attained some better skills and powers, one has only a temporary feeling of satisfaction and success. The moment the child can see something bigger and better beyond where he is at the moment, he again feels inferior, unfulfilled or incomplete. The entire process starts again, a process that leads from inferiority to efforts for new attainments, to achievement of the new level (either symbolically or actually), to recognition of a still higher level, and hence to the inevitable feeling of inferiority once again. This, said Adler, is the stuff of life. The feeling of inferiority introduced at birth is what keeps man living through the ages. Biologically and psychologically he inherits the feeling of inferiority. This drive to achieve and become was taken up as a core theme in the humanist phenomenological approach of Rogers and Maslow. The frustration of the self-assertion need can stem from three sources according to Adler, i.e. organ inferiority, neglect and spoiling.

Organ inferiority (physical defect)

Like Freud, Adler noted that man turns to illness to solve certain non-physical problems. The complaints and syndromes which Adler studied were not associated with the actual condition of the organic system of the patients. Out of these experiences Adler evolved a theory which he referred to as organ inferiority. Compensation for an inferior organ frequently determined the style of life and the manner in which the human would strive for superiority in life: individuals with physical deficiencies often exercise prodigiously to overcome them and attain unbelievable success. For example:

> Demosthenes though a bad stutterer, trained himself to speak and became the greatest orator of Greece; Beethoven became deaf though remained a brilliant composer; many famous painters have suffered from eye defects. (Pickford was able to write a book on colour vision defective art students.) F. D. Roosevelt vigorously pursued a political career after poliomyelitis. Governor Wallace in Alabama is another contemporary example, a permanent cripple in an invalid chair, while the late Sir Douglas Bader overcame the loss of both legs to perform many heroic deeds in World War II.

Organ inferiority was interpreted too as a device used to evade painful and insurmountable tasks as the individual conceived them within his personal frame of reference. A potentially weak organ would come to man's rescue whenever the pressures of life became too strong for him to surmount. If the striving for superiority became blocked or the goal remained totally inaccessible to the individual, he could seek solace and excuse his inferiority by claiming sickness of the weak organ. Thus, some businessmen in highly competitive and pressure-racked occupations develop ulcers, others develop migraine headaches, and still others find solace in sinus difficulties or asthmatic problems, or any type of organic breakdown which allows them to rationalize failure or withdraw from failure-producing situations. The inferior organ, of course, varies from individual to individual.

Neglect

Whether somebody actually was neglected in early childhood or only thinks he was neglected, hated, unwanted or too ugly to be loved, all have the same harmful effect. The subjective evaluation one has of the facts, rather than the facts themselves, matters most. This point has been picked up by self concept theorists and researchers who emphasize the effects of the person's evaluation of his body image in behaviour.

Spoiling

Adler considered spoiling means pampering a child so as to produce dependency. Many spoilt people get on very well in life as long as their path is smooth. As soon as there is an obstacle they fail, because they have never learned to use their own abilities. They do not know that life involves the overcoming of difficulties. As they are not aware that they suffer only from a lack of training, they understandably believe in their own lack of ability and dare not solve problems by themselves.

Adler felt very strongly that the pampered and indulged child is a psychological cripple headed for a life utterly lacking in true superiority of self. He was vehement in his disapproval of parents or any figures of authority who allow the child to be petted and pampered. Yielding too often to the wishes of the child, he felt, deprives the child of the invaluable opportunity to exercise and develop a feeling of superiority within self. Adler's condemnation was directed toward the parents. When a human being has nothing to struggle for because all hurdles have been removed or minimized, he cannot possibly learn how to surmount the hurdles he is forced to meet later in life. The essential relationship between inferiority and superiority is subverted by the artificial superiority supplied by the well-meaning parents. Adler considered the pampered personality the scourge of society. Innumerable times he spoke out against the egocentric demands of the pampered person whose style of life revolves around taking from others to achieve a false superiority, rather than developing within himself the great struggle to emerge from inferiority to superiority.

In summary then, man creates a style of life out of the physical, psychological and social conditions under which he develops. Adler suggested that there are four main lines to attack frustration of the self-assertion drive.

(1) Frontal assault –   a 'small person takes physical exercise, e.g. many weight lifters, 'Mr Atlas', were originally rather puny.

(2) Compensation –   accept the handicap and look for success in another field.

(3) Escape   –   daydream or produce psychosomatic illness, or defence mechanism. One can gain personal power by these means, e.g. in illness you can be judged by more lenient standards. Many neurotic forms of behaviour manifest themselves in this category. The 'Billy Liar' technique is escapism.

(4) Concealment –   hide the frustration under a superiority complex. This is shown in the exaggerated demands an individual makes on himself and on others. They depreciate others to savour their own superiority; the strongest expression of a Superiority Complex is power striving. The deeply hidden doubts in their abilities drives the power strivers on to prove always to themselves and others that they are superior, and never allows them any rest. As they strive towards the goal of personal power and superiority over others, they can never be satisfied.

Style of life

But whatever way we habitually tend to deal with life's frustrations is our style of life according to Adler. Style of life is the way we behave. It is unconscious and created to deal with frustration and inferiority, aimed at the goal of superiority. It develops out of the way we are treated as a child; all children meet denial from parent and nature but all want acceptance; achievement and assertion become, therefore, a style of life and an unconscious strategy to ensure success to prevent inferiority feelings. All neurosis and maladjustment is due to 'wrong' style of life. The task of Adler's psychotherapy is to make a person understand his style, to bring it to the level of awareness.

    This life-style is unique and distinguishes one single individual from all others. To understand the life-style one has to discover the goal towards which an individual is striving. Adler saw a human being always in movement towards his life-goal; from a minus position to a plus position. This striving is not so much influenced by the facts as by the opinion the person has of the facts. The individual does not relate himself to the world in a predetermined manner. He relates himself according to his own interpretation of himself and of his problems. He sees everything from his own self-created perspective. To help patients who have an erroneous opinion to get insight and thus to change their life-style is one of the most important tasks of Adlerian psychotherapy.

Each human being's style of life is unique. No two human beings could have identical styles of life. At least two forces produce a unique style of life for each individual. The first is the individual's heredity. The second force is the variant environment. Since no two human beings can occupy the same space at the same time, the environment for each must, therefore, be different. Even Siamese twins do not look at themselves from the viewpoint of the other. With different environments and different inherited systems, no two human beings can be expected to behave in the same way. To the Freudian, sexuality is the *sine qua non* of all men's behaviour. To the Adlerian, sexuality may or may not be the *sine qua non* of any man's behaviour. It would depend upon his individual style of life. Despite the fact that each life is unique, Adler believed there are certain strong threads which are common to people. Each person has the same goals which he hopes to reach but the paths to these goals are always different. Therefore, his behaviour on the way to these goals is always dissimilar; however, the mainsprings of action are always feelings of inferiority and superiority.

Just as there is consistency in everyone's feelings of inferiority and superiority, so there is a tremendous amount of consistency within one person's style of life. The style of life frequently prescribes a singular interpretative quality for all of the experiences that a human being may encounter. The individual whose style of life revolves around feelings of neglect and being unloved interprets all his experiences from that frame of reference. Activities which are not subject to such interpretation are ignored or twisted into forms appropriate to the desired interpretation. The unloved child feels that all human contacts substantiate his role of being unloved; contacts with people who do give him love prove that that is what life might be for him if he were not unloved. The individual whose style of life centres on feelings of aggression and power considers any display of counterpower a challenge to self, while displays of co-operation or weakness indicate his own strength. It is a strongly interpretative and bonding agent, it controls all actions of life in a determined way. It continues to operate throughout life and remains constant to its core. It is the sole unifying force in life.

From birth to about the age of 5 or 6 years, the style of life is becoming fixed. Based on the inherited capacities of the child and equally important, on the child's use and interpretation of these capacities, the style of life is being formed during these years – and, according to Adler, it rarely changes.

It is far easier to continue in the old and known style, which becomes more mechanical and fixed through the years, than to change. Adler felt so strongly about the formative years in man's childhood that he wrote volumes about educational methods. He was one of the very first to establish child guidance clinics. He also directed a great deal of energy to improving schools, and in particular to educating parents to the risks involved in faulty early childhood training.

Physical disability is highly instrumental in formulating the style of life. Some children with organic weaknesses never surmount their inferiority feelings, and succumb to a style of life defeated and subjected to all the perils of existence. Other children (and many biographies remind us of this) compensate so strongly for an inferior organic weakness that they achieve a degree of superiority far beyond what one might expect from their otherwise normal talents. Examples may be found everywhere. Small-statured people who themselves consider their size an organic defect, although society may not, can be found to have gained out-standing success – if success is the correct word for such as the Hitlers, Mussolinis, and Napoleons of the world!

Masculine protest

Women as well as children are liable to frustration of self-assertion. Adler studied the role of females in Victorian patriarchal society – (is it still the view today that men are the norm and women the deviates?). Freud neglected females in his theory but Adler realised that half the world was female.

Women's resentment and inferiority create the masculine protest. There are two aspects to it:

(1) competitiveness and aggression to men. Through over-compensation they become bad bosses when in power, as those who believe themselves underprivileged cannot assume the virtues of overdogs when unsure of themselves.
(2) overplay role of women, e.g. deliberately appear stereotypically brainless and helpless thus gain by insincerity and cunning.

The common element in (1) and (2) is the overvaluing of the male role, created by our culture pattern. This can occur in men too, for those,

(1) ill-treated in childhood demanding excessive power in adulthood – overcompensation, and
(2) weak, unable to uphold male role act as hen-pecked husband, or dress as women.

Social interest principle

Starting from his initial interest in the assertive characteristics of the human being as an inferiority-to-superiority-driven personality exhibiting a style of life and creative self progression, Adler expanded his theory in 1929 to proclaim that man is also socially interested, a universal interest. This contact with other human beings, Adler stated, is an automatic condition. Man has to be brought up by man just as definitely as he has to be born out of man. Adler reasoned that care of the child must make an impression upon him and that the impression is most logically one that the world is good and that one helps one's fellow man.

Gradually, the predisposition toward other persons is educated into a concern for the welfare of other persons. Being reared by socialized animals turns the baby into a socialized animal. Through elementary school experiences, the child begins to identify with social groups of his own. Through identification, empathy, and co-operation he discovers that a unique reciprocity exists within the world: Help others as you may need help yourself in achieving superiority.

Because man never fully achieves superiority (as soon as one goal is reached the next one beckons), he retains a feeling of inadequacy. The feeling is universal and thus becomes a common bond between men. Held to others by bonds of inadequacy, man trusts that a strong and perfect society can help him achieve for himself a fuller feeling of superiority. The style of life and its more encompassing creative self now incorporate a principle of social interest that permeates his behaviour throughout life.

PSYCHOTHERAPY METHOD

Adler's aim is to make the person conscious of his style of life and replace it by a better one. He employed three methods to study the style of life.

Earliest childhood memories

It doesn't matter if it is true or not. Many people produce lists of child-hood grievances which indicate their views on life. Memories are interpreted according to mood and feeling in the present. First memories allow a deep insight into the human mind. What a person selects out of the multitude of memories indicates on what his interest is still focused. As Adler argues, recalling a danger or an accident, or a punishment, shows great inclination to look at the hostile side of life. The recollection of the birth of a brother or sister shows a retained sense of having been dethroned. The remembrance of the first day in kindergarten or school shows the great impression made by a new experience. The recollection of illness or death is often connected with fear, but more often with the desire to face these dangers better equipped as a doctor or nurse. The recollection of a country holiday with the mother, or the mention of certain persons as mother, father, grandparents in a friendly atmosphere shows preference for these people and the exclusion of others. Recollections of one's own misdeeds, such as theft or lies or sexual vagaries, shows the endeavour to avoid such misdemeanours in the future. First memories reveal distinctly different trends, visual, auditory or motor; these can help in the discovery of the cause of failures in certain subjects at school, or of a mistaken choice of occupation. They aid in helping the individual to select a profession which better suits his preparation for life.

Place in family

Adler made sweeping statements; no tests were conducted, but he was the first to realize that all children in a family do not have the same psychological environment. According to Adler,

(1) The only child thinks people will do what it wants.
(2) The eldest child defends his privileged position for all time, and is a supporter of authority and status quo.
(3) The second born has a pacemaker and tries to keep up to the eldest and outstrip him if possible. He is radical, rebellious, authoritarian.
(4) The youngest always gets much attention and affection from the rest. He is never dethroned and will expect all to be done for him and will struggle to keep up with the rest. All or none attitude – if unsuccessful will give up altogether.
(5) The only girl in family of boys is looked down on or becomes a tomboy to conform to the masculine ideal.
(6) The only boy in a family of girls is petted or ganged up on.
(7) Each position in a family has its unique aspects.

Study of dreams

He regarded symbolism as an attempt to solve some present problem relevant to the style of life. It produces an illusory picture of how to succeed in disregard of the logic of the situation, e.g. flying symbolizes the wish to overcome something without trying, and missing a train is the desire to let trouble pass by. Symbols are not sexual like Freud's, but like Freud he fails to realize dreams express tears as well as wishes. Adler has difficulty in saying why the dream is symbolized as he makes no use of repression.

Adlerian psychotherapy has three main aspects, (1) establishing contact with the patient, (2) elucidating his life-style and (3) encouraging and developing his social interest.

The psychotherapist best establishes contact by maintaining an unchanging friendly attitude. Adlerians approach the client on a non-authoritarian basis and never force him. In order to elucidate the life-style the client is allowed to speak freely. Usually he starts by talking about his present problems. Many find it difficult to talk at all. And this is where from the very beginning encouragement plays an important role. Although the therapist might recognize the life-style early on in the treatment, he should postpone giving his opinion until the client feels able to interpret with him. Gradually his dreams, first memories and his family constellation are interpreted, and his personality is revealed in his thinking and feeling in his movements and actions. He is encouraged to find his real goal.

The current general tendency is to blame parents for the children's difficulties. In contrast, Adlerian psychotherapy helps the client to overcome his bitterness about this. The attitude towards the parents is linked with difficulties which have arisen through the position in the birth order. Even intelligent clients may think they are stupid, because they have grown up in the shade of a very intelligent brother or sister. How much jealousy in later life can be traced back to an often wrong assumption that a sibling is or was preferred? Far from provoking or enlarging feelings of guilt, which lower the self-valuation, Adlerians raise the client's self-esteem. He gets insight into the discrepancy between the facts and his erroneous self-valuation, by the therapist's stressing of his former or present achievements which show he does have abilities. Adlerian psychotherapists emphasize how much more could he achieve, if he gave up his self-limitation.

With the growing self-esteem of the client, the therapist will find it easier to enlarge his social interest. It is not enough to bring him into the company of others, the therapist has first to help him to realize his links with other human beings and rouse his wish to make contact with others. Adlerian therapists are not content with the mere disappearance of the symptoms but only consider the client cured when besides losing these symptoms he strives towards a constructive goal, takes responsibility, courageously solves his problems and acts as a fellow human being.

EVALUATION

Adlerian methods, although very thorough, involve on the whole a short period of time. Adlerian psychotherapy appears valuable for any who have doubts in themselves and cannot cope with life's problems. Such worry is often based in a wrong interpretation of themselves and of the events in which they are part. Adler's approach provides a means of re-learning and establishing a more valid assessment and life-style. It has been suggested that Adlerian psychotherapy can succeed in helping anti-social adolescents to turn into individuals with social interest.

By emphasizing the person's attempt to overcome uncomfortable feelings, he focused attention on ego defences and the adaptive functions of the ego. Adler was arguably the first therapist to consider character structure and the whole person as the proper province for dynamic therapy. Furthermore, he considered the future goals one set for oneself as crucial guiding aspects of one's life. Thus, Adler, like many modern therapists, emphasized the purposive nature of behaviour.

Many Adlerian concepts are part of the layman's general vocabulary, e.g. inferiority complex, striving for superiority. This theory is a down to earth and valuable corrective to Freud's wilder flights of fancy, and this therapy is very valuable for children, and emphasized the importance of social relationships whereas Freud neglected this aspect. However, its comprehensibility has been a source of criticism, for it makes the theory appear superficial and simplistic.

Adler was simultaneously pessimistic and optimistic. Inferiority feelings were inevitable, and thus the neurotic struggle to overcome them also was inevitable. On the other hand, he felt that persons were more malleable and changeable than Freud thought, and the constructive social changes would lead to less debilitating parent–child interactions. Adler was a committed socialist who felt that in order to be healthy a person needed to be unselfishly committed to the good of others, a quality he called 'social interest'. He was in reality the first humanist psycho-therapist providing a bridge between psychoanalysis and phenomen-ology. Underlying his work there is the belief that man has a chance to be better and move forward and upward in life, ameliorate his problems and in general become more adjusted to the life process.

Further reading

Fordham, F. (1953). *An Introduction to Jungian Psychology*. (Harmondsworth: Penguin)
Hall, C. S. and Nordby, V. J. (1974). *A Primer of Jungian Psychology*. (London: Croom Helm)
Orgler, H. (1963). *Alfred Adler*. (London: Sidgwick & Jackson)
Storr, A. (1973). *Jung*. (London: Fontana)

Chapter 4

PRIMAL THERAPY

THEORY

Primal therapy is the brainchild of Arthur Janov (1970). Originally a Freudian psychoanalyst, he claims that patients need to recreate the pain of the birth trauma in order to release themselves from neurosis. He believes that neurosis consists of a warded-off, actual Pain that contains all of an individual's infantile hurts and wrongs. The neurosis is composed of (1) the symbolic attempts a person makes to shun his Pain – the defences – and (2) the chronic state of tension set going as a result of this state of affairs. It is a therapy that bases itself on the unbearable pain of infantile emotional trauma. Like Freud, Janov sees the neurotic as a person struggling with unsolved problems from childhood.

The pain experienced by the child as a sense of being intensely hurt or wronged has been traced by Janov, to what he regards as the first trauma, that of birth. Freud (1926) himself had proposed that the 'trauma' of birth was the prototype of traumatic neuroses. This idea was elaborated by another of Freud's early followers, Rank (1929), who thought that the sudden expulsion from the protecting environment of the womb constituted a trauma which was the precursor of all later experiences of anxiety, and believed that many patients were seeking to re-experience their birth. Leboyer (1977), an obstetrician, has recently drawn attention to the sudden impinging of harsh and violent stimulation on the neonate at birth. The maternity ward can be a kaleidoscope of glaring lights, jangling noises, and sudden movement. Leboyer has introduced quieter and less traumatic methods, which include putting mother and child into immediate physical contact with each other. While still controversial, these ideas have a natural appeal to many obstetricians and paediatricians, and are nearer to the normal practice of most midwives doing

65

home deliveries. There have been reports that minimization of the traumatic separation of mother and infant, and their early re-introduction, foster subsequent 'bonding' between them. Is this a timely reassertion of human values in the face of excessive hospital technology?

Janov's theory lacks two essential Freudian ingredients – repression and infantile sexuality. Janov postulates only one troublesome event – awareness that the parents do not love the child. The theoretical strategy focuses on this particular conflict, the cutting off of feelings experienced as a young child in response to an accumulation of hurts and rejections on the part of the parents. The major primal scene results from the build-up of such small hurts. Eventually the hurts make sense to the child as indications that the parents do not like the child as he is. The recognition of this fact is so traumatic that the child cuts off the feelings and develops an unreal self that protects the child from knowing he or she is suffering. However, the pain associated with these hurts, the primal pain, still exists and continues to manifest itself in everyday life in subtle ways. The neurotic symptoms express the pain. The hurt lies very deep, and neither verbal insight nor superficial tinkering with support, drugs, group pressure or existential awareness will reach it. But it is there and once the defences are down it is really felt and screamed out for the first time, and psychological health will ensue.

TREATMENT

In primal therapy the therapist probes and attacks the defences and confronts the client to help him or her re-experience the pain. This experience of the pain is called a primal. One indication that a person is experiencing a primal is the primal scream, the release of the primal pain that was stored up from childhood.

The therapeutic approach is intense. The patient is given a written set of instructions in advance which defines the terms of the therapy. Included is the directive 'Do exactly as the therapist says. In no case will any harm be allowed to come to you . . .' The patient is told to stay in a hotel and remove himself from regular pursuits for 3 weeks, to abstain from all drugs, sex and other tension-reducing diversions, and to give himself entirely over to the treatment for this period. During this intense phase of the therapy the patient has one open-ended session each day and is the only patient of the therapist for the whole period. Sessions generally last from 2–3 hours each and stop when the therapist decides the client can't take any more. In each session the therapist works actively towards a specific goal (in contrast to having the client free-associate): to get the client to express his deepest feelings towards his parents. And this he eventually does, with baby-talk and screams of violent pain. Everything else is forbidden – dealing with current life situations, explanations of behaviour, exploration of fantasy and, most significantly, feelings towards the therapist.

After completing the three-week intensive phase, the client returns to normal life while continuing his treatment for another 6 months or so with a Primal Group. This is a group very unlike those that have formed the traditional fabric of group therapy. There is virtually no group activity such as communication, interaction, intimacy and power. The people in the group have as little to do with each other as possible. The group thus becomes a backdrop rather than a direct instrument of change.

EVALUATION

Remarkable results have been claimed for primal therapy; and whether these are due to the purging of venomous feelings, as Janov claims, or to a rather more subtle process akin to religious conversion, there is no doubt of its power. The fact that very few people can be treated at a time, and only those who can make a prior commitment to devote 3 weeks exclusively to treatment, creates something of a drawback. But this has to be set against the brevity of the treatment process, compared to the considerably greater long-term investment in time and expense involved in traditional analysis.

Since primal therapy goes so much further than earlier forms of therapy in the direction of religious conversion, it should only be considered by those who want to undergo extremes of experience and to drastically experiment with their lives.

Primal therapy is less likely to be of benefit to people who have problems that require complex judgements about the real world for their solution. Further, people who are particularly suggestible, or those who are emotionally fragile for whatever reason, are placing themselves in positions of risk in emotionally demanding therapies of this sort.

Attaching so much importance to the birth trauma appears quite reductionist, we all have to be born, but we don't all manifest neuroses. Yet there are clients with a history of early trauma who experience a need to scream in therapy, and, in a regressed state, some do appear to experience birth-like bodily sensations. Although there have been reports of dramatic cures from severe neurosis and psychosomatic states following guided re-experience of birth (Lake, 1978), we cannot take them as proof of a causal connection.

Further reading

Janov, A. (1970). *The Primal Scream.* (New York: Dell Publishing Co)

Section III
BEHAVIOURIST APPROACHES

Chapter 5

BEHAVIOUR THERAPY: AN OVERVIEW

INTRODUCTION

Behaviour therapy has as its goal the change or removal of a client's symptoms, usually concentrating upon the directly observable manifestations of behaviour. It is generally held by behaviour therapists that the methods of treatment which they employ derive from theories of learning and conditioning – though there is nowadays a tendency to broaden the behavioural approach to include some apparently successful strategies, which have more doubtful connections with such theories and are, in consequence, referred to as 'behaviour modification' procedures.

Exponents of behaviour modification regard neurotic behaviour purely as a learned pattern of behaviour which is inappropriate and maladaptive. It has to be unlearned, with more adaptive behaviour learned in its place. This is a clear contradiction of the psychoanalytical approach which would regard such neurotic behavioural manifestations as symptoms of underlying mental conflict (a medical model).

Until fairly recently, psychoanalytical theories and the treatments based upon them were virtually unchallenged. Such theories stemmed mainly from the work of Freud, whose teachings gave impetus to a number of breakaway movements which still preserved many of the basic options elaborated by him. The emphasis in such ideas and treatments, however, was clinical and philosophical rather than scientific and experimental, and evidence upon which complex theories about the nature of psychological disturbance was based, had been gathered without proper control and safeguards. This led Eysenck to observe that this reverses the usual procedure of science by attempting to deduce facts and laws from the process of treatment itself. Ordinarily we would expect that theory and practice would evolve from careful, painstaking experimental investigations. In sharp contrast the study of learning and conditioning has been essentially experimental and the theories have evolved from many laboratory studies characterized by scientific orthodoxy. In addition, a further fundamental problem of the psychoanalytical theories has been that of setting up testable deductions. Psychoanalytical ideas are not commonly formulated in such a way that they can be tested with a view to seeing whether they are palpably false or consistent with the results of an experiment.

Eysenck points out that the term 'Behaviour Therapy' is of fairly recent origin, but the techniques of behaviour therapy have a long history. There have been sporadic attempts to apply learning principles to the treatment of maladaptive behaviour since the early 1920s. In the decade following J. B. Watson's famous demonstration that some fears commonly found in children were learned by a conditioning process, there were many isolated instances of therapists using conditioning techniques to eradicate such fears. However, it was not until the late 1950s and early 1960s that a growing dissatisfaction with the results of traditional therapy fuelled by Eysenck's critical papers (see Chapter 21) caused psychologists to look again more closely at this early work.

There are two further objections to psychoanalysis as a preferred mode of treatment. Firstly, it is expensive in terms of skilled manpower. It would be economically impossible to provide the number of analysts needed to deal with the community's problems. Secondly, it is rarely offered to people presenting antisocial disorders, such as delinquency, bullying or destructive behaviour. Yet many of the problems causing most unhappiness in the community as a whole are centred on antisocial behaviour. Behaviour therapy on the other hand is generally of short duration and quite effective with antisocial disorders. The fundamental tenet of behaviour therapy is that behaviour disorders are learned behaviours that are maladaptive in the life of the individual; they are not caused by unconscious conflict, lack of insight, lack of positive regard or any other such concept. In other words, a maladaptive behaviour (e.g. a symptom) is itself the disorder, and it is not a manifestation of a more basic, underlying disturbance. All behaviour is lawful, and unadaptive behaviour is learned and unlearned according to the same principles as adaptive behaviour. In fact behaviour therapists would claim that psychotherapeutic change occurs in both dynamic and humanistic therapies because of unrecognized and unsystematic applications of the same learning principles applied in behaviour therapy.

Behaviour therapists point out that while insight, or self-knowledge, is a worthwhile goal, it does not ensure behaviour change. Often we understand why we behave as we do in a certain situation without being able to change the behaviour. If you are unusually timid about speaking up in group situations you may be able to trace this fear to a number of past events – your father criticized your opinions whenever you expressed them, your mother made a point of correcting your grammar, you had little experience in public speaking during secondary school because you were afraid to compete with your older brother who was captain of the debating team. But understanding these reasons behind your fear probably will not make it easier for you to contribute to class discussion.

Unlike most treatment approaches, behaviour therapy was not founded by a single person. Naturally, certain theorists have made major contributions. Perhaps the most noteworthy are B. F. Skinner and Joseph Wolpe and Albert Bandura. The history of behaviour therapy and its relation to behavioural psychology in the United States begins, in large measure, with John B. Watson (1879–1958), the 'father' of the behaviourist movement, who coined the term 'behaviourism'. While performing certain animal experiments as a doctoral student at the University of Chicago, Watson noted that some data could be verified reliably by other psychologists (e.g. overt acts), whereas other data could not be so verified (e.g. the supposed mental state of the animal). Watson theorized that introspection was a faulty method *per se*, and he urged that scientific psychological research be limited to observing overt acts. Because he focused on observable behaviour, he called himself a 'behaviourist'. Watson wrote, 'The rule or measuring rod which the behaviourist puts in front of him always is: Can I describe this bit of behaviour in terms of "stimulus and response"? (1924, 6)'. Watson is responsible for the following noteworthy evangelical statement.

> I should like to go one step further now and say, 'Give me a dozen healthy infants, well-formed, and my own specified world to bring them up in and I'll guarantee to take anyone at random and train him to become any type of specialist I might select – doctor, lawyer, artist, merchant-chief and, yes, even beggar-man and thief, regardless of his talents, penchants, tendencies, abilities, vocations, and the race of his ancestors.' (1924, p. 104)

Persons were seen as infinitely malleable if only they would learn the proper stimulus–response sequences. The psychotherapeutic ramifications of such a view are self-evident. A. A. Lazarus was the first person to use the terms behaviour therapy and behaviour therapist in a scientific journal article published in 1958. Also in that year Joseph Wolpe published his book '*Psychotherapy by Reciprocal Inhibition*', which may fairly be said to be the first on behaviour therapy. Behaviour therapy, as the name suggests, helps people solve their psychological problems by teaching them new and more effective ways of behaving. The term can be misleading, as many behaviour therapists also help clients deal with disturbing emotions or thoughts. But even when dealing with thoughts and emotions, the behaviour therapist's approach differs from the psychotherapist's approach. The basic difference is that the behaviour therapist sets up specific treatment objectives, usually stated in terms of the client's behaviour. For example, take the case of a client who drinks too much and would like to change. A psychoanalyst would see the drinking behaviour as a symptom of underlying conflict, probably related to deep-seated sexual or aggressive feelings. The goal of treatment would be to help the client gain insight into the conflict, which would lead to a major change in personality. With a more healthy personality, presumably the client would have less need to drink. A client-centred therapist would view the drinking behaviour as symptomatic of a basic incongruity in the client's personality. The treatment goal would be to provide an atmosphere of understanding and acceptance so that the client could experience growth, self-acceptance, and congruence. A Gestalt therapist might see the drinking as reflecting a general lack of self-awareness, and so treatment would be designed to increase awareness. Following such a personality change, the client's desire to drink presumably would be reduced.

In contrast, a behaviour therapist would not view the excessive drinking as a symptom of some deep-seated disorder in the client's personality. Instead a behaviour therapist would view the drinking as the problem itself and would attempt to deal with it directly, using one or more behaviour therapy techniques. For instance, the therapist might have the client imagine vomiting after taking a drink, or teach the client to use deep muscle relaxation instead of alcohol to reduce anxiety. The therapist might also teach the client to control thoughts that usually lead to drinking, such as 'I really could use a drink.' Note that treatment attacks the drinking directly, rather than attempting to reduce drinking by modifying the client's basic personality.

A tentative definition of behaviour therapy has been adopted by the Association for the Advancement of Behaviour Therapy. Although this definition would not be accepted by all behaviour therapists, it does represent an attempt to reflect the broad scope of present behaviour therapy.

Behaviour therapy involves primarily the application of principles derived from research in experimental and social psychology for the alleviation of human suffering and the enhancement of human functioning. Behaviour therapy emphasizes a systematic evaluation of the effectiveness of these applications. Behaviour therapy involves environmental change and social interaction rather than the direct alteration of bodily processes by biological procedures. The aim is primarily educational. The techniques facilitate improved self-control. In the conduct of behaviour therapy, a contractual agreement is usually negotiated, in which mutually agreeable goals and procedures are specified. Responsible practitioners using behavioural approaches are guided by generally accepted ethical principles. (Franks and Wilson, 1975)

Yates (1975) holds that the distinguishing feature of behaviour therapy is the over-riding concern with the experimental investigation of each individual case. No matter how 'standard' a technique might be, its application to an individual requires unique modifications. These modifications are made in accordance with the experimental findings, and the effects of the 'treatment' on the patient are likewise experimentally validated.

Behaviour therapists are agreed that the focus of their attention is on the actual behaviour of the client. They require detailed behavioural descriptions of what the client (or society) is complaining of. For example, a mother may complain that her 4-year-old is 'jealous' of her younger brother. The behaviour therapist will immediately ask, 'How does she show her "jealousy"? How often does she show this behaviour', 'What do you do when she shows this behaviour', and so on. Vague, everyday descriptions of behaviour such as 'jealous', 'scared', 'destructive' are translated in this way into precise operational behavioural descriptions. Having obtained a description of the presenting complaint (and a history of its development as far as can be re-constructed), the behaviour therapist will then try to pinpoint events in the immediate environment which are either maintaining the undesirable behaviour or are preventing the client from learning a new mode of adjustment. In doing so, the therapist is guided by his knowledge of the literature on the ways in which behaviour is learned and maintained. The efficacy of the treatment is then evaluated to demonstrate improvement.

Derived partially, but not totally, from the behaviourist learning principles, a variety of techniques such as systematic desensitization, flooding, modelling, aversion therapy and operant conditioning have been found to be extremely effective in producing more adaptive behaviour in particular areas. Fear (phobic) and anxiety states can be effectively reduced by the first three techniques while undesired antisocial or immoral behaviour can be removed by aversion therapy, with a wide range of possible applications evident for operant conditioning. In all these situations the general approach of behaviour modification is to enable the subject to learn adaptive behaviour patterns he never learned originally or to unlearn maladaptive behaviours.

An interest in the modification of behaviour is certainly not confined to clinicians involved in the treatment of psychological disorders. Such an objective is shared by many, including educationalists, advertising agencies, politicians, and so on.

THE TECHNIQUES

Behaviour therapy of all types basically proceeds in five stages: analysis of the maladaptive behaviour, choice of technique, preparation of the client for the treatment, the application of the treatment technique chosen and evaluation of the treatment. A careful systematic analysis of the client's behaviour is crucial to the success of behaviour therapy. Clients often come to therapy unclear about exactly what is troubling them; it is rare that a client can articulate a highly specific, focused problem. The behaviour therapist, therefore, must help the client pinpoint exactly which behaviour pattern needs changing and which variables in his or her life seem to be causing the maladaptive behaviour. Goldfried and Davison (1976) have identified four types of variables that need to be considered: stimulus antecedents (the environmental determinants), organismic variables (the intrapersonal variables, e.g. client expectations and client physiological states such as fatigue) response variables (the situation-specific maladaptive behavioural response, 'including information on duration, frequency persuasiveness, and intensity') and consequent variables (the environmental response to an emitted behaviour).

Although there is no substitute for direct observation of the maladaptive behaviour in order to perform a careful behavioural analysis, such observation is often impractical and the behaviour therapist must rely mainly on the clinical interview. It is necessary, therefore, that behaviour therapists, as well as dynamic and humanistic therapists, be skilled interviewers. In addition to the interview, behaviour therapists may also use other methods such as questionnaires and outside informants to gather information. When the behavioural assessment is complete, the therapist should have clearly identified the maladaptive behaviour to be changed and the variables that cause it.

Having identified the target of the therapy, the behaviour therapist then selects the most appropriate technique to change the behaviour. Unlike most other types of therapists, behaviour therapists have a wide range of techniques from which to choose their treatment programme.

The third step in behaviour therapy is to prepare the client for the treatment. Often, the rationale of a technique must be explained, or preparatory 'homework assignments' must be given, or the ground rules for a technique must be explained. Whatever preparation is required, including insuring that the client's expectations are realistic, it must be carried out. Fourth, the actual technique is applied, and finally an evaluation of the outcome is conducted. All steps are clearly part of the same therapeutic programme and all may overlap. Behavioural assessment, choice or modification of technique, and preparation are all continuing processes that do not cease once a treatment begins. Furthermore, preparation and treatment may be blended into one process. Part of the technique application may involve homework assignments and self-observation on the client's part. At all times, the behaviour therapist is alert to new behavioural data that might indicate a need for modification or change in technique.

The behaviourist emphasis on the psychological as opposed to the psychoanalytic quasi-disease model of abnormal behaviour has the following consequences:

(1) Abnormal behaviour that is not a function of specific brain dysfunction or biochemical disturbance is assumed to be governed by the same principles that regulate normal behaviour.

(2) Many types of abnormal behaviour formerly regarded as illnesses in themselves, or as signs and symptoms of illness, are better construed as non-pathological 'problems of living' (e.g. neurotic reactions, various forms of sexual deviance, and conduct disorders).

(3) Most abnormal behaviour is assumed to be acquired and maintained in the same manner as normal behaviour; and it can be modified by the application of behavioural procedures.

(4) Behavioural assessments emphasize the current determinants of behaviour rather than the *post hoc* analysis of possible historical antecedents.

Specificity is the hallmark of behavioural assessment and treatment, and it is assumed that the person is best understood and described by what he or she does in particular situations. Hence:

(1) Treatment requires a fine-grain analysis of the problem into components or sub-parts and is targeted at these components specifically and systematically.

(2) Treatment strategies are tailored to the particular problems of the person concerned.

Further reading

Bandura, A. (1969). *Behavior Modification.* (New York: Holt, Rinehart and Winston)

Bolles, R. C. (1975). *Learning Theory.* (New York: Holt, Rinehart and Winston)

Lieberman, D. (1974). *Learning and the Control of Behavior.* (New York: Holt, Rinehart and Winston)

Rimm, D. C. and Masters, J. C. (1974). *Behavior Therapy: Techniques and Empirical Findings.* (New York: Academic Press)

Skinner, B. F. (1974). *About Behaviourism.* (London: Jonathan Cape)

Ullman, L. P. and Krasner, L. (eds.) (1965). *Case Studies in Behavior Modification.* (New York: Holt, Rinehart and Winston)

Chapter 6

OPERANT CONDITIONING and TOKEN REINFORCEMENT

THEORY

These techniques are straightforward applications of Skinner's (1951) research. Positive reinforcement of desired behaviour increases the probability of its repetition, while the ignoring of unwanted responses leads to their extinction. These techniques have great constructive powers in the management of behaviours. Negative reinforcement and punishment are not usually part of the armoury of the behaviour therapist, as these two techniques have many unfortunate side-effects such as withdrawal, anxiety and the provision of wrong models of behaviour to emulate.

Positive reinforcement can be either material (cigarettes, food, toys, money) or it can be social (attention from others, praise). Only a close study of the recipient's reaction to different reinforcers will tell whether they are appropriate. Reinforcements must be given contingently on the appearance of the desired behaviour if it is to be at all effective. This means that the sweet or the praise is given immediately following the appearance of the behaviour, but at no other time. This very simple principle of positive reinforcement is surprisingly potent in altering behaviour.

Whenever a therapist smiles or nods encouragingly after a client has said something, the therapist is using the important operant principle of reinforcement. The deliberate, carefully thought-out application of such operant principles can help people overcome many kinds of self-defeating behaviours.

Some examples of behaviour modification by positive reinforcement and extinction:

(1) Elimination of the psychotic responses of a male schizophrenic who called himself King and was immersed in the royal role. Nurses were instructed to reward him with attention, social approval and rewards (e.g. cigarettes, conversation) only when he talked normally and to ignore him when his delusions of royalty were manifested. The frequence of such delusions decreased dramatically.

(2) Elimination of a child's tantrums and severe crying episodes at bedtime simply by having the parents stay out of the bedroom after the child was put to bed (Extinction). Previously the child had cried and screamed until a parent returned to his room (positive reinforcement for screaming) and the parents had developed a pattern of staying with the child until he fell asleep.

(3) Getting a patient to feed herself, instead of demanding spoon feeding by a nurse. The patient wanted to stay clean and neat, so the nurse was instructed always to spill some food on the patient during spoon feeding. In effect, the patient was taught, 'If you want to stay neat, you will have to feed yourself'. If self-feeding occurred, the nurse reinforced this with praise and social attention.

Operant conditioning involves a rejection of the medical or disease model of human behavioural dysfunction, which assumes some underlying causes of unacceptable behaviour which themselves must be eradicated before that behaviour can change: the operant viewpoint argues that a direct attack upon the behaviour itself can produce all the alterations in external behaviour and internal state which are needed.

The contrast between the two viewpoints may be illustrated by the example of the disordered speech of schizophrenic patients. Where this abnormality is found it is often regarded as part of a disease process and therefore not amenable to modification until the illness has been cured or has remitted. Ullman *et al.* (1964), however, were able to demonstrate that the bizarre verbalizations of schizophrenic patients can be made more normal using reinforcements contingent upon speech. The method involved providing social reward (a nod, a smile, or an encouraging 'mmhm-hmm') when acceptable talk was emitted, but withholding such 'rewards' when peculiar utterances were heard. Positive reinforcement (often tokens) combined with extinction procedures have been mainly employed in schools and hospitals.

PROCEDURE

Whatever the behaviour to be learned, the procedure, in crude outline, involves seven steps:

(1) specify unacceptable behaviour
(2) identify the target (desired) behaviour
(3) obtain pre-treatment baseline of occurrences of unacceptable behaviour
(4) select rewards appropriate to the recipient
(5) whenever the target behaviour occurs, reward it promptly and consistently, though initially shaping by successive approximations will be involved;
(6) Whenever undesirable behaviour occurs ignore it (remember, even punishment can be rewarding to the person receiving such attention!)
(7) evaluate subject's behaviour against pre-treatment baseline

In school contexts

Behaviour modification in school tends to be aimed at keeping children from doing the kind of things that irritate teachers. The assumption is that if pupils 'behave' they will learn more. This is a doubtful assumption, but one that is accepted generally without question. Table 1 lists some of the behaviours teachers can either maintain or modify by the use of appropriate techniques.

A number of successful outcomes using operant conditioning in the classroom have been reported. In a study by Becker, Madsen, Arnold and Thomas (1976), the effects of behaviour modification techniques used by the teacher on ten disruptive children was examined. A typical child was Alice who sulked a lot, sat in her chair moving her hands and legs or sucking her thumb. Before the experiment observers had rated the incidence of her disruptive behaviour, defining 'disruptive' behaviours as those which interfered with classroom learning, violated rules for permissible behaviour established by the teacher and/or reflected particular behaviour a teacher wanted to change. In Alice's case, disruptive behaviour had been noticed in about 50 per cent of the observations made over periods of 20 minutes a day for 5 weeks.

For the experimental procedure Alice's teacher was given specific instructions together with necessary training and support, concerning her reactions to Alice's disruptive behaviour. Some of the instructions were common to all the children in the study. For example, the teacher was told to ignore behaviours that interfered with learning or teaching, unless a

Table 1 Stimulus events and examples of positive reinforcers, extinction and negative reinforcers commonly used

Behaviour	Positive reinforcer (maintains behaviour)	Negative reinforcer (stops behaviour temporarily)	Extinction process (removes behaviour completely)
Talking without permission	Answering, or threatening without following through maintains talking without permission	Punishing as promised (e.g. removing privileges or having student leave group)	Not answering or taking any notice stops this unwanted behaviour
Correctly answering question	Saying immediately 'That is right' encourages further participation	Not commending student discourages further participation interest	Ignoring responses discourages participation
Failing to have required equipment (pens, ruler etc.)	Allowing student to borrow, maintains lax habits	Not allowing borrowing and/or giving failing daily marks promotes adherence to requirements	Ignoring responses encourages adherence to requirements

Disrespectful acts towards teacher	Entering into verbal argument with student or giving lecture on bad manners may maintain behaviour	rapidly punishing without verbal interchange temporarily removes behaviour	Ignoring behaviour extinguishes behaviour
Inappropriate verbal behaviour towards another student	Ignoring it or merely disapproving verbally	Immediate social isolation without verbal interchange	
Turning in extra relevant work	Approval and public acknowledgement	Accusing student of trying to curry favour etc.	Failing to give any approval
Consistently not paying attention to directions and asking that they be repeated	Repeating directions OR mildly scolding the child likely maintains behaviour	Continuing with instructions	Ignoring child

child was being hurt by another and to give praise and attention to behaviours that facilitated learning, at the same time telling the child why he was being praised by using such phrases as 'I like the way you're working quietly, that's the way I like to see you work' and 'Good job! You're doing fine'. There were special rules for Alice. For example, the teacher was told to praise her for sitting in her chair and concentrating on her work, for using her hands for things other than sucking and for attending to directions given by the teacher or to communications from other students. Alice's behaviour was observed for a period of 8 weeks during which the teacher carried out these instructions. During this period the incidence of deviant behaviour in the observation periods, as rated by observers, dropped from 50 per cent to around 20 per cent and stayed at this reduced level; in other words Alice's disruptive behaviour was very considerably reduced.

All but one of the ten children studied in this experiment made similar improvements, and it is unlikely that all these changes were due to chance. Originally, disruptive behaviour occurred in the ten elementary school children on 62 per cent of the occasions on which they were observed. When a teacher followed the instructions specified by the experimenters, the figure dropped to 29 per cent. A particular technique found effective when a child was disruptive, was to ignore the mis-behaviour but, at the same time, praise a child who was behaving in a manner compatible with learning, i.e. combine extinction with positive reinforcement.

In another study, (Orme and Purnell, 1968) of a chaotic classroom in a Boston, Mass., ghetto, the existing behaviour of the 8–9 year olds included: tearing-up papers, throwing books, singing, yelling, taking the desks apart and running out of the classroom. Some idea of the gravity of the situation is given by the fact that, in a 20 minute period, one of the two teachers noted that every child had been struck by another child at least once. When the children were fighting the teacher was only able to restrain two or three pupils at a time and the others would fight on un-restrained – a nightmare situation by any standards.

The instructions given to the teachers in this experiment were similar to those used in the previous study. At first a child might be praised whenever he was simply sitting with his hand up, since it is difficult to fight in this position. At a later stage the teacher would reserve his praise or encouragement for behaviour that was more positively appropriate for learning. Deviant or disruptive behaviour was simply ignored, except when it seemed likely that physical damage would occur to a child. An additional feature of the experiment was that good behaviour could earn points which could be saved and exchanged for tangible rewards. The children used the points to buy articles such as candy and balloons or they could save a large number of points and purchase various experiences judged to be both attractive to the children and educationally valuable such as a ship-building project and field trips to interesting museums. Thus, appropriate behaviour earned the children not only the teacher's praise and encouragement but material rewards as well. This is often termed a token economy.

The results were just as striking as those of the previous experiment. Before the experimental changes, observers' ratings of the children's behaviour using video tapes, produced by a small hidden camera in the classroom, showed that children, on average, spent around 40 or 50 per cent of their time in behaviour that appeared inappropriate for learning. Under the experimental system, the average incidence of disruptive behaviour dropped to about 20 per cent. Various categories of behaviour were observed and all of those judged to be appropriate for learning rose, whereas all the inappropriate or disruptive categories decreased. So, again, the teachers were able to help to produce the sort of classroom atmosphere in which communication and learning is likely to occur.

Schools have long used systems whereby students accumulated points for good behaviour. The points could then be turned in for some material reward. Psychologists have taken over this idea but have preferred to award tokens rather than points. In schools one of the interesting findings is that the token economy may have the effect of reducing the attention of the student to academic matters, perhaps because the student becomes preoccupied with the mechanics of winning tokens, rather than with the acquisition of what he is supposed to learn. Although behaviour modification psychologists suggest that as behaviour improves the token system can be phased out and the naturally occurring reinforcers can be expected to maintain behaviour, there is virtually no evidence available that this happens or can be made to happen. There is little evidence that any improvement in behaviour generalized to other situations becomes a part of the individual's performance.

Levine and Fasnacht (1974) have summarized some fascinating research showing that the use of tokens reduces interest in the academic task. If given a set of problems to solve, human beings will continue, in varying degrees, to continue to solve these problems of their own accord. However, if solving the initial problems is accompanied by a reward not intrinsic to the task, they spend less time, later, solving the problems of their own initiative. This same review also cites studies in which persons performing problem solving tasks produced more creative solutions when no material incentives were offered for their performance. Levine and Fasnacht conclude with the warning, 'Tokens do lead to powerful learning, but the learning may, in fact, be token' (p. 820).

A further problem is that what is positively reinforcing for one person may not be an acceptable one for another, e.g. some children respond well to public praise, others would fight shy of it and respond far better to extra play time and so on. Thus the teacher has to employ his choice of reinforcement sensitively to each individual. With a token economy of course the child can exchange the tokens for his chosen reinforcement, e.g. sweets, a book or a trip out.

In health contexts

The field of medicine has also provided a context for the application of token economies. Patients in mental hospitals often develop what is called 'institutional neurosis': they lose interest in the world and the people around them; they develop hallucinations and fantasies; and they become quarrelsome, resentful and hostile. Institutional neurosis appears to be caused at least in part by the fact that in most hospitals, patients are often treated like children or helpless invalids. That is the patients are 'given' everything they might need by the 'authority figures' in charge. Under these conditions it is little wonder that a rather child-like dependency on the staff develops in the patients.

Behavioural psychologists believe that the best cure for institutional neurosis is making the patient take as much responsibility for his or her improvement as possible. In the money economy that operates in the world outside the hospital, one must typically work to live. Our social system rewards us for 'good' work behaviour with money that can be spent on food, clothing and shelter. If those of us who live in the money economy perform poorly or refuse to work we may very well starve. In contrast, mental hospitals typically operate on a free economy. That is, the patients are given whatever they need merely by asking for it. In fact, the worse they behave, the more attention and help they usually receive; this maintains their patient role dependent behaviour. Behaviourists take the view that, within the hospital economy, it is the patient's 'job' to get well as quickly as possible. Patients should be rewarded for each sign of improvement by receiving 'tokens' that can be traded in for physical pleasures (such as candy, cosmetics, cigarettes, clothes, magazines and records) or special privileges (better jobs in the hospital, going to movies and visits home). In a token economy, therapy usually consists of having the staff reinforce 'socially approved' or 'healthy' behaviours, e.g. conversing normally with staff, and ignoring inappropriate or 'insane' behaviours, e.g. talking in a disturbed fashion. Each patient is encouraged to decide what rewards he or she wants to work for; the patient is then given the tokens as visible evidence that progress is being made toward these chosen goals.

At their best, token economies can lead to rather remarkable changes in the behaviour patterns of certain types of clients – particularly in those who are depressed, withdrawn, immobile or antisocial. There are several reasons for these successes.

(1) Before the token economy can be instituted, the hospital staff must first think about those types of patient behaviours they wish to see increased and those they wish to see decreased in frequency – a type of psychological analysis that few institutional staffs would ordinarily engage in. In short, the staff must decide ahead of time – in very objective terms – what they will consider a 'cure' to be.

(2) The use of tokens forces the staff to focus on healthy behaviours rather than primarily paying attention to those things the patients are doing wrong. Nurses and ward attendants soon learn that many of their patients are more capable of showing improvement than perhaps the staff had thought possible.

(3) Staff members are encouraged to spend more time with the patients than before, since the behavioural therapist can measure the number of staff–patient contacts by monitoring the number of tokens each staff member gives out. The use of tokens also ensures that these interactions will be primarily 'rewarding' rather than 'punishing'.

(4) Individual therapy programmes can be worked out so that each patient in the economy is rewarded primarily for improvement in those 'healthy behaviours' that he or she is most deficient in. Therapy is thus more 'individualized' than it might be in many hospitals.

(5) Both the behavioural therapist and, more important, the patient have a day-by-day record of the patient's improvement – that is, the number of tokens earned. The patient thus gains a greater control over the speed of his or her recovery than is possible in most other institutional milieus.

In one American study, when the operant conditioning programme commenced, 65 per cent of patients in the ward were incontinent, half wore little or no clothing and half could not feed themselves. At the end of the year's training programme, 82 per cent were dry, and 91 per cent completely able to dress themselves without help (Foxx and Azrin, 1973). The Stanley Royd Hospital at Wakefield, UK, experimented with the token economy system for a group of schizophrenics. The results showed that while the token economy had little or no effect on their clinical symptoms, the patients did show considerable improvement in social behaviour. They started to look after themselves, participate in group activities and in the running of the ward. But these improvements were not solely due to the use of tokens, because a group who received tokens immediately they produced desirable behaviour showed similar improvement to a group which received only social approval ('Well done!' etc.) with tokens issued the next day. It would seem that the cause of the improvement is more appropriately located elsewhere. The social approval given where normal behaviour was emitted, the structured and more stimulating daily programme of activities and the higher ratio of nurses to patients all probably contributed to the improvement.

As important as the changes in the behaviour of the patients were the attitudes of the nursing staff. Used to being unable to do more than feed their patients and keep them from injuring themselves and others, the nurses on the token economy ward now found that they were able to help the patients and could see a real improvement as a result of their efforts. Consequently, they were willing to accept the increased demands made upon them that the token economy required.

One of the best-known examples of response-shaping with human subjects is the treatment devised by Lovaas (1966) in order to train six mute autistic children to communicate verbally. The positive reinforcements used in this study consisted of both food and social approval (e.g. 'Good boy!'). Initially the patients were reinforced for emitting any sounds whatsoever at any time. Then, when the frequency of sound production had reached an acceptable level, reinforcement was made more difficult to obtain by making it contingent upon responses produced immediately following an utterance by the therapist. When a subject had learned to do this, rewards were only provided when the sound approximated to that emitted by the therapist. As progress continued to be made, objects corresponding to the words were introduced and the external provided verbal cues gradually faded out. By the end of the programme, these previously non-communicating children were able not only to name simple objects but, also, to string certain words together in a meaningful fashion. The technique of shaping played a very vital role in this treatment.

While operant techniques such as token economies do not provide cures, they do, at least, offer a way of avoiding or eliminating those behaviours which occur because of inappropriate or non-existent schedules of reinforcement that have characterized the grossly understaffed chronic schizophrenic and geriatric wards.

However, Cullen, Hattersley and Tennant (1977) state that the decision to establish a token economy in an institutional setting may be influenced by factors other than the behaviour of the patients. Some of the obvious factors are: (1) increasing the prestige of the institutions, (2) the desire of behaviour modifiers to practise their 'art' and (3) a confusion between controlling the behaviours of patients for the smooth running of the establishment and facilitating rehabilitation.

These factors often lead to the use of the token economy technique in inappropriate settings, and to the initial choice of the least appropriate populations within the institutions, e.g. the 'worst' ward in the establishment of a rehabilitative procedure. Hence the removal of the token treatment conditions often results in the loss of treatment effects (Kazdin and Bootzin, 1972), and generalization of these new responses to environmental conditions beyond the token programme requires to be well planned if such responses are to be maintained in the absence of tokens. Allyon and Azrin (1969), in their pioneering work in this field, attempted to deal with this problem with their 'Relevance of Behaviour Rule' which states 'Teach only those behaviours that will continue to be reinforced after training'. Where a movement of individuals to another environmental setting is not intended it is clear that the token economy could become a permanent feature and be effective in improving management procedures. However, where some degree of rehabilitation into the community is the aim, a careful consideration of the eventual maintaining environment and its similarity to the token environment would be necessary before training began. Thus in one major token economy study, by Atthowe and Krasner (1968), approximately half of the patients who had improved sufficiently to warrant discharge from the hospital, required readmission within a year of discharge. Even where the nature of the in-patient treatment has been extensive and concentrated on such real-life skills as problem-solving, decision-making and self-management (Fairweather, 1964), the rates of rehospitalization have been discouraging. It is estimated that roughly 70 per cent of chronic patients who are discharged from mental hospitals return within 18 months regardless of the type of treatment they received while hospitalized (Fairweather and Simon, 1963).

Although token systems may be advantageous both in establishing and maintaining new patterns of behaviour, their use requires fading as everyday performance characteristics are more closely approximated. The main advantages of token economies are that the technique is good at teaching simple social skills to patients, and in preventing institutional neurosis. A token economy also forces staff to consider their specific objectives for particular patients. The criticism most often raised against the token economy is that it is mechanistic and dehumanizing because it focuses on observable behaviours – on symptoms – rather than on underlying, dynamic psychological problems. From the intra-psychic viewpoint this criticism has considerable merit. The behavioural changes that the token economies do bring about, however, seem to be very reliable (repeatable).

Other applications of positive reinforcement

Anorexia nervosa

A dangerous condition of self-imposed starvation, anorexia nervosa, has been successfully treated with behaviour modification techniques. This disorder usually affects intelligent young women, and patients have been known to die from it. Doctors generally have assumed that anorexia nervosa is a physiological condition, and have sometimes prescribed tube feeding to prevent the death of the patient. Garfinkel, Kline, and Stancer (1973) among others, boldly assumed that the disorder is primarily psychological or behavioural, rather than physiological. Accordingly, they treated five women who had been hospitalized for the condition by rewarding them for weight gains. The rewards included weekend passes and the opportunity to socialize with friends. By the end of the treatment almost all of the patients' weight loss had been regained.

BIOFEEDBACK

Biofeedback is the general name for the training techniques that enable some physiological responses to be brought under voluntary control, such as heart rate and blood pressure. It is the same as operant conditioning but is concerned with the conditioning of responses controlled by the autonomic nervous system; this was once thought to be incapable of voluntary control but it is now accepted that it can be overridden. Until the work of Miller (1969) it had been assumed that psychosomatic disorders such as migraine, certain types of dermatitis, duodenal ulcers and hypertension could not be dealt with by direct methods. However, the findings that certain visceral responses can be shaped in a similar manner to more overt types of behaviour has led to frequent attempts to use operant conditioning with a whole variety of autonomic responses. Biofeedback techniques give subjects information about changes within their own bodies that are normally beyond their awareness. For example, changes in heart rate may be monitored mechanically and electrically. Engel (1972) has reported that people with high blood pressure were trained to lower their blood pressure. The patient watches a visual display of his blood pressure and he is requested to increase or decrease his 'score'. The visual material is also transformed into an auditory signal which informs him of increases and decreases (reinforcement). The patient eventually uses the sound to monitor his performance. He can also be requested to think of calm and drowsy situations to lower the pressure and these thoughts eventually come to condition the pressure.

Patients can produce reductions in systolic blood pressure of around 10 per cent. Reinforcements may be of several different types. Money, praise, self-congratulations and the avoidance of shock have all proved to be effective reinforcers in these types of situations.

Biofeedback training has not been limited to the conditioning of blood pressure and heart rate. Such 'involuntary' responses as electrical activity of the brain, skin temperature, salivation, vomiting and tension headaches may also be affected by biofeedback techniques (Blanchard and Young, 1974). The electromyograph (EMG), which gives precise information as to the degree of tension in specific groups of muscles, has been employed to eliminate those 'nervous headaches' which arise through overactivity of the fontalis.

The EMG has also been used for direct muscle retraining in patients with diminished or absent muscle activity as the result of strokes, spinal damage or other crippling lesions. A number of studies with such patients have shown considerable gains in muscle activity as the result of including biofeedback as part of therapy (Basmajian and Hatch, 1979). Although it is not usually possible to disentangle the particular contribution of bio-feedback the evidence is still quite heartening, and it is significant that physiotherapists are showing an increased interest in the use of biofeed-back for work with this type of patient.

Another application of EEG biofeedback has been with epileptic patients (Sterman and Friar, 1972). This has involved training epileptic patients to increase the amount sensorimotor rhythm found in the EEG. This rhythm is one in the range 12–14 Hz, found over the sensorimotor cortex, and has been found to counteract epileptic fits in some way. It is not clear how this comes about but training epileptics to produce this and other rhythms can have beneficial effects.

From this limited account of biofeedback it can be seen that it offers a novel and interesting approach to the treatment of many clinical problems. In particular it seems to be dealing with a number of physiological problems which may be thought of as stress-related. One particularly interesting aspect of biofeedback is that the patient plays a very active role in the therapeutic process and is primarily responsible for bringing about the changes.

Biofeedback may turn out to have very important repercussions in medicine and be a vital application of operant conditioning. However, it is still too soon to evaluate this approach and the applications of biofeedback are rather controversial. Even Miller (1972) is sceptical of some of his results, and some of the reported results may be due to a placebo or a Hawthorne effect rather than biofeedback itself.

SELF-REGULATION OR SELF-REINFORCEMENT

Another source of reinforcement are the thoughts and feelings of the person themselves. Internal or self-reinforcement is as effective for some clients as external reinforcement. Since client and therapist seldom meet more than once a week, it is to the client's advantage to learn to control or regulate his or her own behaviour, so that progress can be made outside of the therapy hour. Moreover, if people feel they are responsible for their own improvement, they are more likely to maintain such gains. Self-regulation involves monitoring, or observing, one's own behaviour and using various techniques – self-reinforcement, self-punishment, controlling stimulus conditions or developing incompatible responses – to change the maladaptive behaviour. Monitoring one's behaviour consists of keeping a careful record of the kinds of stimuli or situations that elicit the maladaptive behaviour, and the kinds of responses that are incompatible with it. For example, a person concerned with dependency on alcohol would note the kinds of situations in which he or she is most tempted to drink, and try to control such situations or devise a response that is incompatible with drinking. A man who finds it hard not to join his co-workers for a liquid lunch might plan to eat lunch at his desk, thus avoiding the situation. If he is tempted to relax with a drink on arriving home from work, he might substitute a game of tennis or a jog around the block as a means of relieving tension. Both of these activities would be incompatible with drinking.

Self-reinforcement is rewarding yourself immediately for achieving a specific goal – such as praising yourself, watching a favourite TV programme, telephoning a friend or eating a favourite food. Self-punishment means that you arrange some aversive consequence for failing to achieve a goal – such as depriving yourself of something you enjoy (not watching a favourite TV programme) or making yourself do some unpleasant task (cleaning your room). Depending on the kind of behaviour you want to change, various combinations of self-reinforcement, self-punishment, or controlling of stimuli and responses might be used.

For example:
A programme for the self-regulation of eating.

Self-monitoring

Daily log – Keep a detailed record of everything you eat. Note amount eaten, type of food and caloric value, time of day and the circumstances of eating. This record will establish the caloric intake that is maintaining your present weight. It will also help to identify the stimuli that elicit and reinforce your eating behaviour.

Weight chart – Decide how much you want to lose and set a weekly goal for weight loss. Your weekly goal should be realistic – between 1 and 2 pounds. Record your weight each day on graph paper. In addition to showing how weight varies with food intake, this visual record will reinforce your dieting efforts as you observe progress toward your goal.

Controlling stimulus conditions
Use these procedures to narrow the range of stimuli associated with eating:

(1)   Eat only at predetermined times, at a specific table, using a special place mat and so forth. Do *not* eat at other times or in other places – for example, while standing in the kitchen.
(2)   Do not combine eating with other activities, such as reading or watching television.
(3)   Keep in the house only those foods that are permitted on your diet.
(4)   Shop for food only after having had a full meal, and buy only those items that are on a previously prepared list.

Modifying actual eating behaviour
Use these procedures to break the chain of responses that make eating automatic:

(1)   Eat very slowly while paying close attention to the food.
(2)   Finish chewing and swallowing before putting more food on the fork.

(3) Put your utensils down for periodic short breaks before continuing to eat.

Developing incompatible responses

When tempted to eat at times other than those specified, find a substitute activity that is incompatible with eating. For example, exercise to music, go for a walk, talk with a friend (preferably one who knows you are dieting), study your diet plan and weight graph noting how much weight you have lost.

Self-reinforcement

Arrange to reward yourself with an activity you enjoy (watching television, reading, planning a shopping trip, visiting a friend) when you have maintained appropriate eating behaviour for a day. Plan larger rewards (for example, buying something you want or a holiday) for a specified amount of weight loss. Self-punishment (other than forgoing a reward) is probably less effective because dieting is a fairly depressing business anyway. But you might decrease the frequency of binge eating by immediately reciting to yourself the aversive consequences or by looking at an unattractive picture of yourself in a swim suit!

Further reading

Ayllon, T. and Azrin, N. (1968). *The Token Economy.* (New York: Appleton-Century-Crofts)

Bandura, A. (1969). *Behavior Modification.* (New York: Holt, Rinehart and Winston)

Danskin, D. and Crow, M. (1981). *Biofeedback.* (Palo Alto: Mayfield)

Gatchel, R. and Price, K. (1979). *Clinical Applications of Biofeedback.* (New York: Pergamon)

Goldfried, M. and Merbaum, M. (1973). *Behavior Change Through Self Control.* (New York: Holt, Rinehart and Winston)

Jehu, D. *et al.* (1972). *Behaviour Modification in Social Work.* (London: Wiley-Interscience)

Kazdin, A. (1975). *Behaviour Modification in Applied Settings.* (London: Irwin Dorsey)

Lazarus, A. (1971). *Behaviour Therapy and Beyond.* (London: McGraw-Hill)

Poteet, J. (1974). *Behaviour Modification.* (London: University of London Press)

Thoreson, C. and Mahoney, M. (1974). *Behavioral Self-Control.* (New York: Holt, Rinehart and Winston)

Ullman, L. and Krasner, L. (eds.) (1965). *Case Studies in Behavioral Modification.* (New York: Holt, Rinehart and Winston)

Chapter 7

SYSTEMATIC DESENSITIZATION

THEORY

Systematic desensitization can be viewed as a 'deconditioning', or a 'counter-conditioning', process. This procedure is very effective in eliminating fears or phobias. The idea is to weaken a maladaptive response by strengthening an incompatible or antagonistic response. For example, relaxation is antagonistic to anxiety; it is difficult to be both relaxed and anxious at the same time. Wolpe (1958), who developed this technique, called this process reciprocal inhibition. Emotional reactions may be classically conditioned. If we consistently experience pleasure in someone's company, then the mere mention of the person's name will set off pleasant feelings. In the same way, fear, anxiety and guilt may also be classically conditioned to stimuli and situations. Two important studies preceded Wolpe's work and provided evidence that phobias are learned and can be removed using learning theory procedures. The first is the case of Albert reported by Watson and Rayner (1920). They provided a classical demonstration of the development of a phobia in a young child. Having first ascertained that it was a neutral object, they presented an 11 month-old boy, Albert, with a white rat to play with. Whenever he reached for the animal the experimenters made a loud noise behind the boy. After only five trials Albert began showing signs of fear in the presence of the white rat. This fear then generalized to similar stimuli such as furry objects, cotton wool and white rabbits. These phobic reactions were still present when Albert was tested 4 months later. The process involved in this demonstration provides a striking illustration of the way in which phobias can develop. The implications of this work are discussed in detail elsewhere (Wolpe and Rachman, 1960). It is sufficient for present purposes to note that this demonstration provided the first model of human neurosis.

The second investigation of importance was that reported by Jones (1924). A 3 year-old boy, Peter, showed fear of white rats, rabbits, fur, cotton wool and other similar objects. Jones treated Peter by de-conditioning methods. It was decided to start on the rabbit phobia as this seemed to be a focus of Peter's fears.

' Peter was gradually introduced to contacts with a rabbit during his daily play period. He was placed in a play group with fearless children and the rabbit was brought into the room for short periods each day. Peter's toleration of the rabbit was gradually improved. The progressive steps observed in the process included: rabbit in cage 12 feet away tolerated . . . in cage 4 feet away tolerated . . . close by in cage tolerated . . . free in room tolerated . . . eventually, fondling rabbit affectionately.'

Another measure employed by Jones involved the use of feeding responses. 'Through the presence of the pleasant stimulus (food) whenever the rabbit was shown, the fear was eliminated gradually in favour of a positive response.'

Using these techniques Jones overcame not only Peter's fear of rabbits but all his associated fears. The follow-up of this case showed no resurgence of the phobia. Like the two little boys above, some people find themselves caught in the grip of extremely strong, apparently irrational, fears. Cases have been reported in which individuals were terrified of such stimuli as illness, social contacts, death, cats, travel, being alone, injection, blood, going insane, pregnancy, medicines and fainting among other things. This is not the mild uneasiness we may all feel in connection with some of those stimuli and situations, these are overwhelming specific fears, called phobias that incapacitate the individual. For example, many people are so fearful of social situations that they can never bring themselves to leave the protection of their homes (agoraphobics).

The deconditioning of fear in humans involves creating

(1) some pleasant condition that counteracts the anxiety so that the organism comes to associate the stimulus situation with pleasure;

(2) a graduated approach to the feared situation. The basic paradigm is:

Early trials

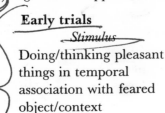

Stimulus		Response
Doing/thinking pleasant things in temporal association with feared object/context	⟶	No anxiety (recipricol inhibition)

Later trials

Stimulus		*Response*
Feared object/context	$\longrightarrow$	No anxiety with toleration of former, feared object/context

This paradigm is of course the basic model of classical conditioning as proposed by Pavlov.

THE TECHNIQUE

The method of systematically desensitizing a person to a feared situation involves first training the individual to relax, and then gradually exposing him or her to the feared situation, either in imagination or in reality. In relaxation training, the individual learns to alternately contract and then relax various muscles, starting for example, with the feet and ankles and proceeding up the body to face and neck muscles. The person learns what it feels like when muscles are truly relaxed (as compared to tense), and to discriminate various degrees of tension. Sometimes drugs and hypnosis are used to help people who cannot otherwise relax.

While the individual is learning to relax, he or she works with the behaviour therapist to construct an anxiety hierarchy, a list of situations or stimuli that make the person feel anxious; the situations are ranked in order from the least anxiety producing to the most fearful. For example, for a woman who is so fearful of interacting with other people that she feels anxious when she leaves the security of her home, the hierarchy might start with a walk to the corner post box. Somewhere around the middle of the list might be a drive to the supermarket. At the top of the list might be a plane trip alone to visit a friend in a distant city. After the woman has learned to relax and the list has been constructed, desensitization begins. She sits with her eyes closed in a comfortable chair while the therapist describes the least anxiety-producing situation to her. If she can imagine herself in the situation without any increase in muscle tension, the therapist proceeds to the next item on the list. If the woman reports any anxiety while visualizing a scene, she concentrates on relaxing, and the same scene is visualized again until all anxiety is neutralized. This process continues through a series of sessions until the situation that originally provoked the most anxiety now elicits only relaxation. Through this method, the woman is systematically desensitized to anxiety-provoking situations by the strengthening of an antagonistic or incompatible response – relaxation.

Although desensitization through visually imagined scenes has been effective in reducing fears or phobias, it is less effective than desensitization through actual encounters with the feared stimuli – which is not surprising. That is, the woman in our hypothetical case would probably lose her fears more rapidly and more permanently if she actually exposed herself to the anxiety-producing situations, in a sequence of graduated steps, and managed to remain calm (Sherman, 1973). When possible, a behaviour therapist tries to combine real life with symbolic desensitization. Systematic desensitization can be divided into four stages:

(1) Preliminaries (history taking etc.).
(2) The client is trained in progressive relaxation.
(3) Hierarchies of phobic stimuli and/or anxiety-provoking situations are constructed and ranked in ascending order of intensity.
(4) The client is required to imagine the phobic stimuli in gradually ascending order, while in a state of deep relaxation.

Table 2 depicts two examples of anxiety (phobic) hierarchies.

Table 2

A. Claustrophobic Series

(1) Being stuck in a lift (The longer the time, the more disturbing)
(2) Being locked in a room (The smaller the room and the longer the time, the more disturbing)
(3) Passing through a tunnel in a railway train (The longer the tunnel, the more disturbing)
(4) Travelling in a lift alone (The greater the distance, the more disturbing)
(5) Travelling in a lift with an operator (The longer the distance, the more disturbing)
(6) On a bus journey (The longer the journey, the more disturbing)
(7) Stuck in a dress with a stuck zipper
(8) Visiting and unable to leave at will (e.g., if engaged in a card game)
(9) Being told of somebody in jail
(10) Reading of miners trapped underground

B. Death Series

(1) Being at a funeral
(2) Being at a house of mourning
(3) The word death
(4) Seeing a funeral procession (The nearer, the more disturbing)
(5) The sight of a dead animal (e.g. a dog)
(6) Driving past a cemetery (The nearer, the more disturbing)

Adapted from Wolpe, J. (1961). The systematic desensitization treatment of neuroses. *J. Nerv. Ment. Dis.* **132**, 189.

When the client is relaxed, the therapist asks him to think about the situation from those listed that produced the least amount of anxiety. If the client is thoroughly relaxed, he will be able to think about the situation without feeling anxiety, since the anxiety will be incompatible with the relaxed state. What usually happens is that the client will not be able to attain sufficient relaxation on his first trials, but slowly the therapist will help him reach the point where he can contemplate the anxiety producing idea in a state of relaxation. Once he has accomplished this he is on the road to being able to think of, and encounter, the anxiety-producing situation without it producing anxiety in him.

Once the weakest of the hierarchical stimuli has been desensitized and no longer elicits fear, the therapist can move up the hierarchy presenting more and more disturbing stimuli, one at a time. In each case, the patient is asked to relax in the presence of the disturbing stimulus. In this manner, a patient may overcome the fear of producing qualities of even the most frightening stimuli. This desensitizing method has been successful with many different phobias (Rachlin, 1976), and sexual dysfunctions (Masters and Johnson, 1966). Each scene or item is presented repeatedly until such time as the patient can tolerate it without experiencing any discomfort. Typically, the therapist will ensure reaching this criterion for each step in the hierarchy before passing to the next one in the list.

EVALUATION

Initially, systematic desensitization was used mainly with monosymptomatic phobias. Difficult, more generalized anxiety of social situations such as is involved in agoraphobia (an intense fear of being out alone in public places) also responds to this form of treatment, although recent studies indicate that 'flooding' (see later) is an even more successful technique.

Reviewing the literature on the efficacy of systematic desensitization, Meyer and Chesser (1970) report success rates ranging from 62 per cent to 100 per cent. The better figures tended to come from studies of monosymptomatic phobias. Agoraphobia was found to respond better to desensitization than to individual or group psychotherapy. One of the obvious advantages of systematic desensitization is that it takes a much shorter time than traditional psychotherapy. Many studies report treatment being successful in as few as ten sessions. Follow-up studies show that gains are maintained and that the removal of the unwanted fear has not resulted in the appearance of new 'symptoms'.

The earliest reports on the use of this method lacked the kind of experimental controls necessary to adequate evaluation. Wolpe's (1958) data, obtained from 210 patients, suffered this defect, and it is difficult to attach significance to his report that about 90 per cent of neurotic patients respond favourably to desensitization. The same may be said of data published by Lazarus (1963) concerning the treatment of 408 neurotic patients. However, what is interesting in this latter study is the differential results obtained with patients suffering from more severe forms of disturbance. Overall, the figure for 'cure' or 'much improved' was 78 per cent, but the same statistic for the severely disturbed group was only 62 per cent; in other words it appears that desensitization works better with milder forms of neurotic disorder than the more severe kinds.

Rachman (1966b) notes that although some psychologists and psychoanalysts had predicted unfavourable side-effects of desensitization, none had been reported. In particular, the expectation that patients would substitute one symptom for another did not materialize. Wolpe and many others believe that these changes are the result of learning to handle disturbing stimuli in a relaxed fashion, that the lack of muscular tension leads to or induces the shift in the patient's attitudes. Other therapists insist that Wolpe has put the cart before the horse, that cognitive changes occur first and thereby allow the client to relax in the presence of the dreaded stimulus. As evidence, these critics cite research suggesting that one need not start at the bottom of the fear hierarchy and work up gradually to the most disturbing item; instead, one can pick items at random and expose the client to them (as long as he or she doesn't become too disturbed by the procedure). Some studies show that purely mental relaxation may be as potent a curative agent as is muscular relaxation. Despite controversy over how and why it works there is a great deal of sound evidence that desensitization treatment works very well indeed (and very speedily) in eliminating the fears of normal – that is, not psychiatrically disturbed – individuals.

Marks and Gelder (1965) conducted a retrospective study which enabled a useful comparison to be made between desensitization therapy and psychotherapy, and the respective contributions which these treatments made to different types of phobic clients. The outcome in general was decidedly favourable to desensitization where phobias other than agoraphobia were concerned, particularly in the period immediately following treatment. For agoraphobias there was little difference between the two treatments given, neither of which appeared to be specially beneficial. Since the mid-1960s a wide range of studies have been conducted, generally successfully on a wide variety of fears among normal and neurotic persons. For example here follow a number of reports of successful desensitization.

Kravetz and Forness (1971) report an experiment with a 6½-year-old boy who could not speak when in the classroom. A desentisization programme of 12 sessions (2 per week) was established. The anxiety-evoking stimulus hierarchy used in this study is presented below.

(1) Reading alone to investigator
(2) Reading alone to room-mate
(3) Reading to two classroom aides (repeated)
(4) Reading to teacher and classroom aides (repeated)
(5) Reading to teacher, classroom aides and small group of classroom peers (repeated)
(6) Reading to entire class
(7) Asking questions or making comments at weekly ward meeting when all patients, teachers and staff were present

This desensitization programme combined with positive reinforcement, was successful in assisting the boy to overcome his fear of verbalizing in the classroom.

Parrino (1971) applied systematic desensitization to reduce the frequency of the grandmal seizures of a 36-year-old man. It was determined by observation that the seizures were triggered by specific anxiety-provoking situations such as:

(1) socializing with fellow patients
(2) meeting persons in authority
(3) initiating conversations with acquaintances
(4) interacting with female patients who were harassing him
(5) hearing family-related material such as his wife's or his child's name.

The desensitization sessions, which lasted for 15 weeks, focussed on the following anxiety-evoking stimulus hierarchy:

(1) a person you would recognize appears in the unit
(2) the acquaintance is having a conversation with a staff member
(3) the acquaintance looks in your direction
(4) the acquaintance and you make eye contact
(5) the acquaintance smiles at you from across the room
(6) the acquaintance starts walking towards you
(7) the acquaintance is getting very close to you
(8) the acquaintance extends his hand to you
(9) you shake hands with the acquaintance
(10) you engage in conversation with the acquaintance.

The subject of this therapeutic intervention returned to full-time employment and remained almost free of seizures.

Marzagao (1972) reported a case study of a 24 year-old woman with a 12 year-old history of kleptomania. This abnormal behaviour was used by the woman to reduce anxiety in specific situations, such as being left alone in a strange setting. A total of 17 desensitization sessions were conducted with the subject during the treatment process. She imagined herself in the following situations;

(1) chatting with girl-friend and making an appointment to study in the home of one of her friends
(2) arriving at the friend's place alone
(3) going into her friend's study and finding her alone
(4) chatting with the friend while awaiting other students
(5) noticing her friend's handbag on the bed
(6) being invited by the friend to go to the dining room to have a snack
(7) refusing the invitation and asking the friend to bring the snack to the study
(8) being alone in the study and making sure of being unobserved
(9) picking up the handbag.

No relapse had occurred 10 months after treatment.

Garvey and Hegrenes (1966) reported a similar study concerning Jimmy, a 10 year-old with school phobia. During treatment the therapist eliminated the child's fear of school by having him approach the school accompanied by the therapist and by proceeding with the following anxiety-evoking stimulus hierarchy;

(1) sitting in the car in front of the school
(2) getting out of the car and approaching the kerb
(3) going to the pavement
(4) going to the bottom of the steps of the school
(5) going to the top of the steps
(6) going to the door
(7) entering the school
(8) approaching the classroom in a certain distance each day down the hall
(9) entering the classroom
(10) being present in the classroom with the teacher
(11) being present in the classroom with the teacher and one or two classmates
(12) being present in the classroom with a full class.

After 20 consecutive daily treatments Jimmy resumed a normal school routine; no return of the phobia was noted during a 2 year follow up study. Before the implementation of this intervention Jimmy had participated in 6 months of traditional psychotherapy without apparent success.

These and other studies employing normal individuals with isolated phobias have certainly confirmed expectations generated by earlier experiments with animals. They show a high success rate in removing such fears, an often remarkable brevity of treatment and a superiority over other methods with which desensitization has been compared. In addition, these investigations lent considerable support to the effectiveness of relaxation as a counter anxiety state, and to special requirement of compiling an 'anxiety hierarchy!' But recent evidence suggests that items from the hierarchy may be presented in any order, with much the same outcome. This is termed 'flooding'.

Flooding

In systematic desensitization, a hierarchy of feared contexts or stimuli are successively worked through, commencing with the least evocative and proceeding in sequence to those that would ordinarily produce strong negative emotions, while the client is in a state of relaxation. However in Flooding the client is 'thrown in at the deep end' and led to re-experience in therapy the original trauma assumed to be responsible for the intense emotional reaction. So instead of proceeding cautiously step by step up the hierarchy, flooding requires the presentation of the most anxiety evoking stimuli initially (Stampfl and Levis, 1967). Flooding is alternatively called implosive therapy. The assumption is that keeping the client in this situation, and preventing him from engaging in his usual escape reactions, allows him to 'discover' that the anticipated traumatic event does not occur, and the anxiety will then extinguish.

One or two early studies (Rachman, 1966b), suggested that this may not be a useful therapy, although Wolpin and Raines (1966) had found the method effective. The technique itself can appear rather startling, since its deliberately conceived purpose is to maximize anxiety associated with the cues to fear. Hogan and Kirchner (1967) for example, treated a group of students for their fear of rats who were asked to imagine the most horrifying scene involving these animals. They were told to imagine that rats were running all over their bodies, getting inside their bodies, gnawing at their organs, and so on. In another context Wolpe (1969) has reported the use of flooding treatment in a dentist who could not give injections to his patients in case they died in his surgery. Therapy involved the vivid portrayal of the dentist giving an injection, withdrawing the syringe, and then observing the patient slump forward, dead. The earliest response of patients to implosion is, not surprisingly, acute distress, but this tends to give place to a calmer state as the 'scene' continues, until all anxiety has disappeared.

However, Wolpe (1969) has pointed out that while some patients benefit greatly from flooding, others fare badly and can become worse.

More recently there has been some suggestion, from experimental studies as well as from clinical practice, that the more severely disturbed patient may be most responsive to implosion. Furthermore, it is thought possible that desensitization and implosion may be useful complementary treatments, dealing with patients of varying degrees of disturbance. For example Meyer et al. (1974) have found that massive exposure to the object of a patient's fear, when combined with other training, can produce excellent results in the severely handicapped obsessional patient. Briefly, they have found that the anxiety such patients experience when brought into contact with some source of imagined 'contamination', can be brought under control if the individual is exposed to contamination and is prevented from either running away or engaging in some ritualistic activity.

However, there are still too few adequately controlled experimental studies of implosive therapy, but clearly it can be quite economic in terms of the therapist's time.

Assertive training

Another kind of response that is antagonistic to anxiety is an approach, or assertive, response. Some people feel anxious in social situations because they don't know how to 'speak up' for what they feel is right, or to 'say no' when others take advantage of them.

Assertive training teaches people to express their feelings and thoughts in a straightforward but socially acceptable manner. According to Wolpe (1958; 1969), being assertive brings two main benefits. First, an assertive person is more effective in dealing with other people, and, therefore, should have more satisfying personal relationships. Second, strange as this may sound, behaving assertively has the effect of making you feel less anxious (Rimm et al., 1974), apparently because it decreases physiological arousal.

By practicing assertive responses – first in role playing with the therapist and then in real-life situations – the individual not only reduces anxiety but also develops more effective coping techniques. The therapist determines the kinds of situations in which the person is passive, and then helps him or her think of and practice some assertive responses that might be effective in those situations. The following situations might be worked through during therapy sessions:

(1) Someone steps in front of you in a queue
(2) A friend asks you to do something you don't want to do
(3) Your boss criticizes you unjustly
(4) You return defective merchandise to a store
(5) You are annoyed by the continual conversation of people behind you in the theatre
(6) The mechanic did an unsatisfactory job of repairing your car
(7) The bus conductor gives you wrong change.

Most people do not enjoy dealing with such situations, but some are so fearful of asserting themselves themselves that they say nothing, and build up feelings of resentment and inadequacy instead. Assertive training involves rehearsing with the therapist effective responses that could be made in such situations and gradually trying them out in real life.

The principal technique in assertive training is called behaviour rehearsal. The client begins by describing a troublesome interpersonal situation such as asking the boss for a raise. The therapist then has the client 'act out' the way he or she usually behaves in such a situation. The therapist points out deficiencies as well as positive features, perhaps noting that the client's voice was not very loud, and that the client avoided eye contact with the therapist, who had assumed the role of the boss. The therapist then proceeds to act out what the therapist considers to be a more appropriate and effective response. The client then acts the situation out again, thus imitating the therapist's response. The procedure continues until both the client and therapist are satisfied with the client's response, and further, the client feels comfortable in making the response. The client and therapist can then go on to another troublesome interpersonal situation.

The description may make assertive training seem easy, but it is one of the most difficult of the behaviour therapy techniques. The reason is that the therapist must be aware of what responses are or are not effective and appropriate in an endless number of interpersonal situations. This takes a lot of experience.

Many research studies (Lange & Jacubowski, 1976) indicate that assertive training is effective. But studies also indicate an important limitation.

Training a person to be assertive in one situation does not generalize or transfer very much to other situations (Rimm & Master, 1974). If you are taught to be more assertive to your employer, don't expect this to generalize to your wife!

Further reading

Wolpe, J. (1958). *Psychotherapy by Reciprocal Inhibition*. (Stanford: Stanford University Press)

Wolpe, J. and Lazarus, A. (1966). *Behaviour Therapy Techniques*. (Oxford: Pergamon)

Chapter 8

MODELLING

THEORY

As we have seen with systematic desensitization, controlled exposure to the phobic situation, either in reality or in imagery and thought, is a valuable component of effective treatment. However, highly phobic individuals are, by definition, reluctant to confront the source of the fears.

Social learning theory accepts traditional learning theory, but it also considers the common-sense observation that persons learn not only by doing, but also by observing behaviour of models (either in the real world, or through various media). It is beyond doubt that completely novel responses can be learned by observation. For instance, it is easier to teach a beginner the forehand stroke in tennis by having her watch a film of a skilled tennis player, rather than by rewarding her after each discrete portion of the stroke is performed. Furthermore, emotional as well as physical responses may be learned through observation. Such common-sense observations which are not explained by traditional learning theory, are the basis of social learning experimentation and theory.

In an important, much cited, experiment, Bandura (1965) demonstrated many of the principles of social learning theory. Nursery-school children were assigned to three groups; each group watched a film in which a model attacked an adult-sized 'Bobo doll' in various specific ways. Children in the first group only saw the model attack the doll; the second group also saw an extra scene in which an adult punished the model for attacking the doll. After seeing the film, each child was placed in a room which contained a 'Bobo doll' and various other toys. There were sufficiently varied toys so that the child could behave like or unlike the model in the film. The child's aggressive behaviour in this situation was recorded through a one-way mirror. The results demonstrated that children who saw the model in the film receive either a reward or no punishment for attacking the doll now responded more aggressively (i.e. imitatively) than did the children who had seen the model punished.

To determine if the children had acquired the ability to imitate the response, whether or not they had performed imitative behaviour when alone, the experimenter returned after a brief isolation period to inform the child that for every imitative response he or she could perform a reward would be given. The results were that in every group the children produced more imitative aggressive behaviour than they had when alone. Thus a person may acquire a new response through observation and learning, even if he or she does not perform that response immediately. Reward and punishment might thus affect a person's performance of the observed response, but it need not affect his acquisition of the responses. In sum, real-life and experimental observation clearly confirm that learning occurs through observation of the behaviour of models.

Observing learning is affected by numerous variables, many of which have been empirically investigated. Hilgard and Bower (1975) summarized a sampling of variables studied by Bandura.

Stimulus properties of the model
(1) The model's age and status relative to that of the subject
    High-status and older models are more imitated
(2) The model's similarity to the subject: Imitation induced in the subject decreases as the model is made more dissimilar to a real person.

Type of behaviour exemplified by the model
(1) The more complex the skills, the poorer the degree of imitation after one observation trial
(2) Hostile or aggressive responses are strongly imitated
(3) Standards of self-reward for good versus bad performances. The subject will adopt self-reward standards similar to those of the model. Also the subject will imitate the type of moral standards exhibited by an adult model. Techniques of self-control can be transmitted in this manner.

Consequences of model's behaviour
(1) Rewarded behaviours of the model are more likely to be imitated than punished or ignored behaviours.

Naturally, a subject can only learn through observation if she pays attention to the model's behaviour. It should be noted that many of the variables listed above, such as subject–model similarity, have an effect on whether or not a subject will pay attention to a model.

Liebert has also suggested that observational learning can be described fruitfully as a three-stage process: exposure, acquisition, and subsequent acceptance of modelled responses. According to Liebert, acceptance occurs if after being exposed to and acquiring modelled responses, 'the observer now employs them or accepts them as a guide for his own action' (in Liebert and Spiegler, 1974, 389–90).

APPLICATION

Modelling has been used successfully to overcome a variety of fears or avoidance behaviours, and to teach new, more adaptive responses. Modelling is often combined with role playing in which the therapist helps the individual rehearse or practice more adaptive behaviours. In the following excerpt a therapist helps a young man overcome his anxieties about asking girls for dates. The young man has been pretending to talk to a girl over the phone and finishes by asking for a date.

> *Client:* By the way (pause) I don't suppose you want to go out Saturday night.
> *Therapist:* Up to actually asking for the date you were very good. However, if I were the girl, I think I might have been a bit offended when you said, 'By the way'. It's like asking her out is pretty casual. Also the way you phrased the question, you are kind of suggesting to her that she doesn't want to go out with you. Pretend for the moment I'm you. Now, how does this sound. There is a movie at the Varsity Theatre this Saturday that I want to see. If you don't have other plans, I'd like very much to take you.
> *Client:* That sounded good. Like you were sure of yourself and like the girl, too.
> *Therapist:* Why don't you try it?
> *Client:* You know that movie at the Varsity? Well, I'd like to go, and I'd like to take you Saturday, if you don't have anything better to do.
> *Therapist:* Well, that certainly was better. Your tone of voice was especially good. But the last line, 'if you don't have anything better to do' sounds like you don't think you have too much to offer. Why not run through it one more time.
> *Client:* I'd like to see the show at the Varsity, Saturday, and if you haven't made other plans, I'd like to take you.
> *Therapist:* Much better. Excellent, in fact. You were confident, forceful and sincere. (Rimm and Masters, 1974, p. 94)

A considerable number of experiments by Bandura and his co-workers suggest that imitation or modelling is a very potent way of learning or adopting new behaviour. For example: Bandura, Grusec and Menlove (1967) have shown that it is possible for children to overcome fears of harmless dogs by watching other children interact with dogs. A related technique, participant modelling, has been very effective in helping certain phobics overcome their fears (Rimm and Medeiros, 1970). Suppose you are afraid of harmless snakes and you seek help from a therapist who decides to use participant modelling. The therapist will begin by approaching a caged (and manageable) harmless snake, and in graduated steps, will open the cage, touch the snake, and handle the snake. You will probably experience some reduction in fear by observing this. Then the therapist will guide you through a similar sequence of behaviours at your own pace – this is why it is called participant modelling. You may find that within an hour, you have effectively conquered this fear of snakes (Bandura, Blanchard and Ritter, 1969). Participant modelling has also been used to overcome fears of high places and of water (Hunziker, 1972).

Bandura, Jeffrey and Wright (1974) demonstrated that participant modelling is successful because it provides a number of 'performance aids' such as prior modelling of the feared activity by the therapist, joint

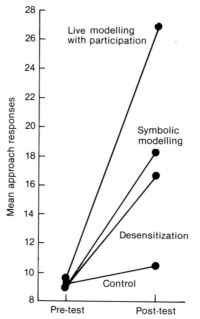

Figure 3 Treatment of snake phobia. The mean number of snake-approach responses made by subjects both before and after receiving behaviour therapy treatment. (After Bandura *et al.*, 1969).

performance of graduated sub-tasks and initial control of the feared situation by the therapist. The greater the degree of supportive performance aids in the participant modelling procedure, the more rapid and marked were the changes in avoidance behaviour and phobic attitudes.

As well as participant modelling (which is often called live modelling), phobic subjects may watch a filmed model engage in the feared activity (often called symbolic modelling), or even rehearse the model's actions in imagination (usually called covert modelling).

Figure 3 compares different levels of effectiveness of various types of treatment.

Modelling has also proved effective in reducing the fears of young children about to be admitted to hospital for operations. Melamed (1977) used a film of a happy, relaxed child accompanied by its parents, entering hospital. Admission procedures, preparation for surgery and return home, were all shown in the film. The child actor was never shown to portray fear or anxiety. This modelling film resulted in significantly lower levels of anxiety in the experimental group than in a control group who saw an unrelated film as measured by palmar sweat pre- and post-operatively.

EVALUATION

The outcome of research has tended to be favourable to modelling procedures, in the sense that fears have shown greater reduction than has been the case using control 'treatments', e.g. superior to desensitization for snake phobia (Bandura *et al.*, 1969), and the benefit has shown generalization to situations and stimuli outside the context in which the experiment has been performed. It has also been found that when symbolic modelling (e.g. seeing a recorded example of an undisturbed person dealing with the phobic object) is supported by participant modelling (where model and subject take part in a live exercise) the improvement is further increased.

However, too little is known about this method and its value with psychiatric patients to be certain about its potential in pathological states. Certainly there is not sufficient evidence to form any clear idea of the comparative efficiency of modelling and other behavioural procedures.

A social learning/imitation model has a ready appeal in terms of explaining the acquisition of abnormalities for which no such personal traumatic event or series of smaller events in combination is evident. The social-learning/imitation model does not need to assume that such events are part of the individual's history.

The account does require that exposure to vicarious learning has taken place and it is notable that a patient sometimes has a parent who had the same fear. Unhappily, of course, opportunities for vicarious learning in the individual's history cannot be easily traced and identified.

Indeed, the modelling explanation of fear acquisition presents a difficult problem: so many fear models – in films, TV and elsewhere – home in upon the individual that perhaps phobias should be a good deal more common than they are. No doubt, the salience of the fear model experience for the individual, the degree to which he can detach himself from that experience and the temperament he brings to the situation, are all relevant considerations here.

However, the importance of Bandura's work is that behaviour may change not just by the reinforcements we receive but can be strongly affected by what we observe. We are strongly influenced by the models around us. Not only do we learn to cope with stress by observing how others around us handle stress, but we can learn new coping styles from our observations. Bandura has accumulated impressive evidence to demonstrate that observing life models (as opposed to filmed models) cope well with situations, that are fearful for the person who is observing, can significantly change that person's ability to cope with the situation in real life. Seeing someone cope with petting a large dog or handling a non-poisonous snake or a difficult social situation can be an effective therapy intervention leading to behaviour change.

Further reading

Bandura, A. (1965). Influence of models' reinforcement contingencies on the acquisition of imitative responses. *J. Pers. Soc. Psychol.*, **1**, 589–595

Bandura, A. (1969). *Principles of Behavior Modification*. (New York: Holt, Rinehart and Winston)

Bandura, A. (1977). *Social Learning Theory*. (Englewood Cliffs: Prentice Hall)

Chapter 9

AVERSION THERAPY

THEORY

This technique is employed for the treatment of behaviour disorders in which the client's behaviour transgresses convention or is immoral, even though it is highly self-rewarding. It is based on Pavlovian classical conditioning. Aversion treatment attempts to do the opposite of desensitization. Desensitization tries to reduce a patient's fearful or unpleasant associations to a situation so that he can enter the situation with equanimity. In contrast, aversion treatment deliberately tries to eliminate certain patterns of behaviour by associating them with unpleasant stimuli. Of course, punishment has been employed in such conditions since time immemorial by parents, teachers and legislators, and even doctors once used ingenious devices of punishment ranging from special twirling stools to machines which doused water on to clients' heads from a height until the client behaviour was altered in the desired direction. Systematic application of aversion in psychiatry began about 20 years ago with the introduction of chemical methods of aversion. Emetic drugs were usually given by injection, to induce vomiting while the client carried out his undesirable behaviour. This procedure was designed to condition the client to feel nausea whenever he subsequently tried to carry out the undesirable behaviour. However, chemical methods of aversion are cumbersome, unpleasant and difficult to administer with any precision, so improved techniques were sought. Electric aversion has begun to replace chemical aversion in the last 5 years as it is safer, less unpleasant, and easier to use.

APPLICATION

Classical conditioning provides the model for aversion therapy, as the

113

undesirable behaviour is linked in treatment to unpleasant experiences. Alcoholism, sexual perversion and drug taking are associated in the treatment with a variety of noxious stimuli, such as electric shocks and emetics so that the response to the unconditioned stimulus also becomes conditioned to the undesirable behaviour.

The basic paradigm is as follows:

Early Trials
    Undesirable behaviour ⟶ Emetic ⟶ Discomfort
Later Trials
    Undesirable behaviour ⟶ Discomfort

Aversion therapy tends to be quite brief, taking perhaps 2 or 3 weeks. However, the unwanted behaviours suppressed by aversion therapy show a great capacity for revival, so, to counteract this tendency to relapse booster' courses of treatment are generally given at suitable intervals in time.

The use of electric shock is well-illustrated in the study by Sylvester and Liversedge (1960) who treated a selection of clients suffering from occupational cramps. Analysis of the difficulties of writer's cramp sufferers revealed the presence of two distinct abnormalities, tremor and muscle spasm, each of which required separate attention.

To deal with the tremor, a metal plate was drilled with holes of graduated size and the patient was required to insert a metal stylus into these, starting with the largest. Any marked tremor would lead to contact between stylus and plate which would complete an electrical circuit resulting in a strong shock being given. This aversive stimulus would lead to avoidance of the aberrant activity (tremor), and the client could then proceed to increase his control using one of the smaller holes.

The aversive stimulus also can be an unpleasant taste or smell – Foreyt and Kennedy (1971) used a nauseating smell in treating obese subjects. In Joseph Cautela's (1967) method of covert sensitization, no actual aversive stimulus is used. Instead, clients imagine aversive consequences after engaging in some undesirable habit. For instance, an overweight person imagines feelings of nausea after eating some forbidden food (Janda & Rimm, 1972). Sometimes the aversive experience may be directly related to the habit itself. When cigarette smokers inhale every 5 or 6 seconds, the experience can be very unpleasant and may result in a reduction in smoking (Lichtenstein et al., 1973).

Not entirely typical of chemically induced aversion, is the use of the drug Scolene (suxamethonium chloride) which produces muscle and respiratory paralysis. Sanderson et al. (1963) have reported on the use of this drug in the treatment of alcoholism; it is injected immediately after the client has looked at and sniffed his chosen drink, and he is allowed to sip a little just before the expected onset of paralysis. The client remains completely conscious while the drug is acting but cannot speak, move or breathe for a minute or so and the experience is very traumatic.

Many reports of aversion therapy have tended to focus upon the sexual problems of individuals, typical of which is that by Blakemore *et al.* (1963). This client was a transvestite who had, since the age of four, derived pleasure from dressing in female clothing. In his twenties, he frequently cross–dressed and appeared publicly, as he described it, as a 'complete woman'. Aversion therapy involved having the client 'dress up' while standing on an electric grid so that, at any time the therapist chose, a shock could be delivered while the patient was engaged in the pleasurable activity. The shock would be given repeatedly until the patient had divested himself of female clothing. Treatment was intensive, five 'trials' of the kind described being given at half-hourly intervals for about 8 hours each day, over a 6 day period. The outcome was successful in this case and remained so over the 6 months of follow up.

Voegtlin, Lemere and their colleagues (1942) have reported on the treatment of more than 4000 cases of alcoholism with a lengthy follow-up inquiry. It is difficult to arrive at any firm conclusion from these investigations which were marked by changes in procedure and developments in technique and so on. However, they report that abstinence from alcohol for periods up to 5 years was found in 50 per cent of cases treated, although this figure had dropped to 13 per cent by the end of 13 years.

This kind of result, obtained by the uncomplicated application of noxious stimulation for a specified type of behaviour (drinking alcohol) points to the relapse over time associated with such therapy. This is where positive reinforcement can play its part. Relapse generally occurs because, after successful treatment, the client returns to his own environment where it is likely two things occur: (1) the newly learned behaviour is not reinforced and is, therefore, extinguished and (2) contemporaneously, old behaviour is strongly rewarded. So, unless 'an old soak' can be weaned away from his former drinking pals and haunts, relapse is inevitable. The answer is to place the client in an environment where he will receive positive reinforcement for maintaining his new behaviour, for example, the 'dried out' alcoholics must be introduced into an AA group. This provides a new set of friends and a new environment where the acceptable alternative behaviour will receive group reinforcement and support. You cannot leave the client on his own after successful removal of the undesirable behaviour, a return to old ways is so easy in former haunts, since conditioning has ceased and extinction will occur anyway without other support and reinforcement.

On its own, aversion therapy does nothing to make the socially desirable alternative behaviours more attractive for the client. For this reason, most therapists nowadays attempt to modify the client's social environment so that newly acquired alternative responses have an opportunity of appearing and being reinforced.

A similar combination of strategies is employed in some aversion therapy treatment of sexual deviancy, a combination which not only enables a client to rid himself of old unwanted behaviours but, also, encourages the growth and development of more acceptable responses, in other words, positive reinforcement. Typical of this tendency is the now common practice of discouraging some forms of sexual deviancy by using electric shocks, while allowing relief from shock when some more appropriate, heterosexual behaviour is performed.

As an example of this, the aversion therapy treatment of a homosexual may involve showing the patient a picture of homosexual activity during which time a strong electric shock is given. At any point in time, the client may be allowed to switch off the slide and, by doing so, terminate the shock. This, in turn, results in the automatic projection of a picture depicting heterosexual activity. In essence, therefore, the situation is one in which homosexual stimuli are 'punished' while heterosexual stimuli are being associated with the escape from the shock (e.g. Feldman and Macculloch, 1965).

Bed wetting or enuresis, has also been analysed in terms of classical conditioning. Normally, bladder tension is the conditioned stimulus or CS that evokes a waking response (the conditioned response or CR). Most children probably learn this CS–CR connection in the following fashion. Bladder tension (CS) is paired with an unconditional stimulus (UCS) such as a wet bed, which causes the child to wake up. Through repeated pairings, the bladder tension (CS) normally acquires the capacity to elicit the waking response. But some children do not learn this CS–CR connection, probably because wetting the bed does not awaken them. Therefore, these children sleep through the bladder tension and wet the bed.

As far back as 1938 (Mowrer, 1964), psychologists were attempting to control enuresis through classical conditioning. They reasoned that, since the CS (bladder tension)–CR (waking) connection has not been learned, it may be established by pairing the CS (bladder tension) with an alternative UCS that elicits the desired waking reponse in a more effective manner.

Mowrer devised an apparatus to help train the child to gain control. He put tiny electrical wires in a thin cloth pad that could go under the bottom sheet on the child's bed. These wires were connected to a loud bell near the head. Whenever the child urinated while asleep, the urine (which is a good electrical conductor) closed the circuit that rang the bell, waking the child up. Although the amount of current involved was so small that the child received no electrical shock to its body, being rudely aroused in the middle of the night was often so distressing that the child's brain often 'learned' to heed the signals coming from the bladder and woke the young person up before an accident could occur. Mowrer's device has been an effective training tool for many children.

Further reading

Cambell, H. and Church, R. M. (eds.) (1969). *Punishment & Aversive Behavior.* (New York: Appleton-Century-Crofts)
Franks, C. (1969). Behavior and its Pavlovian Origins. In Franks, C. (ed.) *Behavior Therapy: Appraisal and Status.* (New York: McGraw-Hill)

Chapter 10

(handwritten margin note)

BEHAVIOUR MODIFICATION – Ⓐ PANACEA OR AN EVIL?

(handwritten margin note: bitter/ine in feel in spee)

Opposition to behaviour modification has often been vitriolic, and the examples in school and hospital already given above may lead some readers to agree with such condemning phrases as 'as nasty as it is naive' (Koestler, 1967), and 'as congenial to an anarchist as to a Nazi' (Chomsky, 1972).

What in general aroused these passions was the belief that applied conditioning theory would produce a society not much different to that portrayed in Aldous Huxley's *Brave New World*. However, a recent flood of operant conditioning studies as applied to environmental problems (e.g. energy consumption and litter) suggests that Skinner's work is not as ill boding for society as was formerly believed (Davey, 1981).

ETHICAL CONSIDERATIONS

Behaviour modification possesses some unique qualities as a social movement (Leung, 1975).

(1) it is action orientated rather than descriptive
(2) it acknowledges the importance of social designation of abnormal behaviour, and
(3) its goals are explicit, open to inspection and this, perhaps, renders it liable to attack.

Any discussion of the ways in which psychological techniques are being used to alter human behaviour will lead inevitably to questions of the morality of such behaviour modification. The whole philosophical issue is complex but some points are worth bringing out.

Ullman (1969) points out that the medical model provides an ethical rationale for treatment by an '*a priori*' standard of 'health' and 'pathology'. Since behaviour modifiers tend to construe abnormality as a result of past history of reinforcement they face ethical decisions with which the medical model has not been confronted. First, if abnormal behaviour is considered learned, the therapists are involved in making, or at least concurring with, a value judgement that some other behaviour would be preferable. They are responsible not only for the cessation of one set of behaviours but also for the behaviours that replace the previous ones. More than that, instead of believing in 'sickness' or 'health', behaviour modification is in sympathy with the idea that the evaluation of abnormal behaviour is usually a societal judgement (Blackman, 1973). The behaviouristic position is primarily a deterministic one, and this is incompatible with the ideal of freedom of choice. This comes into conflict with the legal position of 'freedom' and 'dignity' (Wexler, 1973).

In general, most scientific research has a potential for either good or bad use, to a greater or lesser extent. It is not the psychologists' role to decide on the uses of his discoveries but neither can he reject all responsibility. Since he knows better than most the potential of his findings he should play an active part in attempting to direct any use to which they may be put to the benefit, rather than to the detriment of mankind. The problem of what is of benefit to mankind still remains.

In the case of behaviourist control, visions of a dictatorship described by Orwell (1954) in '*1984*' are easily aroused. Indeed, many regimes with similarities to '*1984*', using a common-sense knowledge of behavioural control, have existed in the past and show no signs of going out of fashion. However, such horrors are better seen as a warning of the dangers of misusing behavioural control than as its necessary and unavoidable end-product. An analogy from biochemistry is that the grotesque results of errors in the testing of thalidomide warn of the dangers of misusing new drugs, but do not cause us to condemn all pharmaceutical research.

The alteration of human behaviour by the application of processes derived from animal learning research in the Skinner box suggests the elimination of the freedom of the individual. In a sense, even for the pigeon in the Skinner box, this is not so. The pigeon does not have to peck the button. We should not confuse the descriptive laws of science – 'This is how things happen' – with the prescriptive laws of a legal system – 'You must do this'. The latter involves compulsion from outside the individual, the former does not. Even so, behavioural control does involve someone else planning what an individual should do.

The amount of freedom considered desirable varies from person to person. Most of us would agree that everyone should be free to hold whatever political views he likes. There would be less agreement on the desirability of the freedom to use others for personal profit. Few would agree with the freedom to murder. The extent to which individual freedom is limited for the benefit of the rest of the population varies from society to society, but limitations are usually imposed without causing general discontent. The extent to which behavioural control is put into practice will depend on the ethics of the existing society.

There are many problems with the concept of freedom. It has led Skinner to write a book entitled *Beyond Freedom and Dignity* (1971), in which he argues that theories about the freedom and dignity of man have developed as a way of escaping and avoiding the aversive control usually exercised by dictators. Ethics based on freedom and dignity help to avert aversive control. However, they also prevent the planning of environments based on positive reinforcement, in which desirable behaviours are shaped and maintained by reinforcers which people would like to receive. Skinner argues that it is necessary to go beyond the concepts of freedom and dignity and develop ethics which are more appropriate to what we know about behaviour.

It is often said that these methods are simply ways of inducing conformity in people, and that manipulation of other persons, as is implied in all behaviouristic methods, is inherently wrong and inhumane. But from birth to the grave man attempts to manipulate others, and is in turn manipulated by them. The baby is 'manipulated' to suck at the mother's breast, and later on to take solid food and come off the mother's breast. The child is 'manipulated' to learn how to read and write, plus all the other things which he needs in order to live happily in society. The adolescent is 'manipulated' to take a job, earn a living and eventually maintain a family. The girl is 'manipulated' into bed by her boyfriend. The voter is 'manipulated' by the politicians whose concern for his welfare is far less apparent after than before the election. We are all 'manipulated' by advertisements to buy this rather than that. Sometimes manipulation is disguised as appeal to reason, usually a not very convincing mask. Wisdom begins with the realization that all social living implies manipulation of one person by another; manipulation is the essence of social living.

Equally important as the fact of manipulation is the motive for manipulation. All manipulation is not bad; without it we would still be animals living in a state of nature – our lives according to Hobbes being nasty, brutish and short. Some kinds of manipulation are obviously of help to the person concerned, e.g. the baby would starve if his mother did not orient his mouth correctly to the breast. Children, as they grow up, often reproach their *laissez-faire* parents, saying: 'Why didn't you make me do that?' when some deficit becomes apparent in their education or upbringing, and which could easily have been dealt with earlier on.

On the other hand, manipulation can obviously also be bad, in the sense that it is used for the interest of the manipulator, rather than of the person manipulated. It seems hardly necessary to give examples, advertising which makes use of natural fears of death, disease, social isolation and other negative feelings for the purpose of selling useless and possibly dangerous drugs.

In short, behaviourist psychology is in exactly the same position as all science, as far as application is concerned; whether it is applied to the benefit or the detriment of mankind, depends on mankind itself, not on the scientists in question. When Rutherford split the atom, he was convinced that this discovery would never be of any practical use. Since then, we have seen this discovery applied to the making of nuclear weapons; we have also seen it applied to the creation of energy urgently needed by mankind to replace the rapidly depleting reserves of natural fuels. We have to learn to look at both sides, and then come to realistic conclusions about the balance in terms of the quality of human life.

Blackman (1973) states that the real issue 'centres on what patterns of behaviour we should seek to control'. Thus this choice of what behaviour to control is guided by the controller's value judgement. Krasner (1969) sees that there is no reason why a behaviour modifier cannot use his own values as the determinant of what is most socially desirable. Miron (1968) makes an equally arbitrary claim that a behaviour modifier should work for the maximum benefit to the patient and to society, giving careful consideration to cases where the two may conflict. What is the solution when the therapist cannot agree with either society or the patient? Skinner (1971) argues that what you do is simply allow those who already control to control more effectively. This implicitly accepts the therapist's position as an 'agent of his employer'.

Skinner (1971, p. 136) believes that 'survival is the only value according to which a culture is eventually to be judged, and any practice that furthers survival has survived value by definition'. In the light of this statement, behaviour modification should aim at the furtherance of the survival of the human species. However, the moral issue still exists. When one is confronted with the hypothetical situation where the survival of A jeopardizes the survival of B, who should be awarded the priority?

When we consider whether we should attempt to control behaviour, it should be remembered that we are influenced by conditioning and learning all the time. Our behaviour is shaped and controlled by the stimuli and reinforcers which occur in our environment. The question at issue is whether this conditioning should be consciously controlled or left to·occur by chance.

There is always an underlying value judgement made that one behaviour is undesirable and another desirable, particularly when aversion therapy is to be applied. Who should make this judgement? Are we right in imposing our values and standards on others? Should the client always give his consent based on his informed judgement before any behavioural modification treatment commences? There are no 'correct' answers to these questions, but we must be aware of such ethical problems and form our own opinions on them. But unquestionably behaviour therapy has much to offer in the treatment of certain types of behaviour problems and is a well-accepted form of treatment. The fear has been expressed that aversion therapy, and positive reinforcement may be employed solely to secure conformity to laws of society and is, in this sense, better suited to the function of the policeman than the therapist. It is of paramount importance to establish that such treatments are in the interests of the individual who is actively seeking change, but this is not always an easy problem for the therapist to decide.

Whether one can have an acceptable treatment which apparently involves the infliction of punishment is yet another issue. Of course the issue is not confined to aversion therapy, for surgery, dentistry, and other therapies frequently involve inflicting considerable amounts of pain. Most likely it is the deliberate and calculated use of pain as a means of obtaining change which some may find unacceptable, and they will point out that the pain of the dentist's drill is a by-product which the dentist does his best to minimize. The ethical arguments often advanced against using aversion therapy certainly carry some weight, and these must be set against the reasoning that, often, no alternative treatments may be available, that the client's strong desire to change must be considered, and that one must presume the integrity of the therapist as is the case in any other treatment endeavour.

One fallacy as regards practising behaviour modification is that only aversive control, coercion and deprivation would arouse public hostility. Wexler (1973) however, argues from the legal point of view that positive controls can be equally troubling. In psychiatric institutions one sometimes wonders whether the idea of requiring patients to work, particularly without standard compensation, is sheer exploitation, labour saving or therapy. This is particularly pertinent to token economies wherein positive reinforcers are given contingent upon the residents' performance of a target behaviour. Therefore daily routines like sweeping the floor are accorded the values of 'therapeutic assignments'. Simple occurrences like refusing to go to the workshop or getting up late in the morning can also mean being unco-operative in therapy.

OTHER PROBLEMS

Practical problems are a further area of difficulty in behaviour modification, just as they are in other treatment procedures. One which the therapist encounters, not infrequently, is that of arranging the changes in behaviours which are effected in the clinical setting to show transfer to the actual life situation of the individual concerned. Relatively few published accounts make any serious reference to the differentiations which an individual may make between behaviour produced under the therapist's gaze and that which may be emitted in the naturalistic setting, yet such problems are not uncommon. Securing the transfer to the real world, and testing out one's capacity to 'cope' in that setting, remain problems.

Some critics have raised serious doubts about the intentions of many of these therapeutic programmes, saying that they are intended to create acquiescence rather than to bring about real therapeutic change. In reply to this it can be seen that increasing the self-help of retarded clients by token reinforcement frees the staff and clients from many time-consuming, menial tasks and allows for a more productive use of the gained time for both groups. Moreover, it is also argued that with schizophrenic patients, such approaches can arrest the social deterioration which is often found in long-stay institutions.

Practical problems often arise within the hospital or clinic settings which abort or disrupt attempts at behaviour modification. It is not uncommon to find that the manipulation of reinforcements in operant conditioning programmes is made difficult by clients who receive unscheduled rewards from friends, relatives or other clients. It is not uncommon to find the alcoholic client, before coming to hospital for treatment has thoughtfully arranged a secret supply of his favourite beverage. It is not untypical that drug-addicted clients should continue to receive supplies from a kindly visiting friend.

However, perhaps one of the most pressing problems is that while desensitization training often liberates the individual to enjoy more of life than before, aversion therapy can create new difficulties for the patient to face. Blocking some behaviour which has afforded satisfaction may leave the individual without any readily available alternatives; the homosexual deprived of his deviant impulse, does not 'naturally' become a well adjusted heterosexually oriented individual, and the alcoholic who has become a non-drinker has lost many friends and is left with an 'occupational' void.

Obviously aversion therapy would be more successful if it were always accompanied by some other type of training which helps the individual to realize other forms of satisfaction which could be available. To some extent recent endeavours in the field have attempted to do just this (e.g. Feldman and Macculloch, 1965).

The part which motivation plays in treatment, and how this may be assessed constitutes another difficulty. It seems very probable, that clients who are pressed to seek treatment by the courts, by marriage partners and the like, do less well than those who seek help of their own volition. These and numerous other technical issues remain serious problems.

It is often said by the critics of behaviour modification theories that there is a serious neglect of 'internal' processes. There is, as a result of the historical origins of these methods, an emphasis upon observable behaviour, and a relative neglect of the inner world of attitudes, thought and emotions. It is also true that many applications of behaviour modification techniques involve a dependence upon little-understood internal processes, such as asking the client to imagine a scene in desensitization or to conjure up a fantasy of sexual activity in the course of aversion therapy. In these circumstances there is a paucity of information concerning what is actually going on in the client's 'mind', and this must be regarded as a serious problem and hazard for current theoretical formulations. Clearly, there must be certain reservations about what is happening when we treat a client by giving electric shocks whenever he reports having a particular fantasy; is his tendency to report fewer fantasies an index of improvement, is it the result of a calculated unwillingness to think about this scene because of the shock which follows or is the subject having the fantasy, but refusing to report it? Finally, the usual criticism of any procedure involving the behavourist tenets of faith is brought against behaviour modification. It is seen as cold, impersonal and mechanistic.

On the other hand the benefits of behaviour therapy have been well documented. For example, Kazdin and Wilson (1978) made a comprehensive analysis of 75 comparative clinical outcome studies. Although few of the studies were sufficiently well designed to allow for unambiguous interpretation results, Kazdin and Wilson were able to extract the following conclusions:

(1) Not a single comparison showed behaviour therapy to be inferior to psychotherapy. Most studies showed behaviour therapy was either

marginally or significantly more effective than the alternative treatment.

(2) No evidence of symptom substitution following behaviour therapy was observed, even in studies explicitly designed to uncover negative side effects. Typical of the findings in this respect is Sloane *et al.'s* (1975) comment:

> 'not a single patient whose original problems had substantially improved reported new symptoms cropping up. On the contrary, assessors had the informal impression that when a patient's primary symptoms improved, he often spontaneously reported improvement of other minor difficulties' (p. 100).

(3) Behaviour therapy is more broadly applicable to the full range of psychological disorders than traditional psychotherapy.

IS THE THEORETICAL RATIONALE IMPORTANT?

Although behaviour modifiers claim that maladjusted behaviour is learned and therefore that learning theory principles can be applied to alter such behaviour, it is questionable in some instances to what extent the therapy is underlain by the principles and empirical relationships discovered in the behaviourist learning theorists' experimental laboratory. London (1972) avers that behaviour therapists employ learning theory simply as a paradigm, analogy and metaphor to guide their approach which is essentially pragmatic. Behaviour therapy is perhaps better regarded as a technological system with a minimum of theoretical rationale, whose only common thread is a commitment to detailed operational analysis of individual problems coupled with a systematic search for techniques that will produce required changes. For example according to London (*op cit*) the link between classical conditioning systematic desensitization is weak. First, it involves the use of language which is uninvolved in classical conditioning. Second, it includes covert imagery a mechanism that has not been studied in conditioning studies. Third, it is subject to successful variations that were not predictable from studies that led to the technique in the first place. Only in positive reinforcement, extinction techniques and token economies can a direct transfer of behaviourist learning theory principles be seen.

What we have seen then is that behaviour modification is a set of techniques based largely on learning theory principles which are employed to alter observable behavioural problems. Maladaptive behaviour is regarded as learned; hence it can be unlearned and new behaviour learned in its place. Positive reinforcement taken from the operant conditioning model has been used to increase the production of desired behaviour. This has been particularly effective and beneficial in aiding geriatric and mentally ill patients to develop acceptable personal and social habits, using tokens as secondary reinforcers. Such techniques combining extinction and positive reinforcement have also been applied effectively in the school setting to modify the behaviour of children with behaviour problems.

Systematic desensitization has been successful with minor fears and phobias. Aversion therapy using emetics or electric shocks removes behaviour that transgresses social convention, such as drug abuse and alcoholism, though reinforcement of the new behaviour is required to prevent relapse. Behaviour modification involves ethical considerations about imposing on others value judgements of what constitutes acceptable behaviour.

Biofeedback appears to offer considerable promise for the alleviation of medical problems such as hypertension and stress related symptoms.

Further reading

Franks, C. and Wilson G. T. (1974). The nature of behavior therapy: recurring problems and issues. In Franks, C. and Wilson, G. T. (eds.) *Ann. Rev. Behav. Ther.* Vol. 2. (New York: Brunner/Mazel)

Franks, C. and Wilson, G. T. (1975). Ethical and related issues in behavior therapy. In Franks, C. and Wilson, G. T. (eds.) *Ann. Rev. Behav. Ther.* Vol. 3 (New York: Brunner/Mazel)

London, P. (1964). *The Modes and Morals of Psychotherapy.* (New York: Holt, Rinehart and Winston)

London, P. (1972). The end of ideology in behavior modification. *Am. Psychol.,* **27,** 913–20

Mahoney, M. *et al.* (1974). Behaviour Modification: delusion or deliverance? In Franks, C. and Wilson, G. T. (eds.) *Ann. Rev. Behav. Ther.* Vol. 2 (New York: Brunner/Mazel)

Marks, I. (1976). The current status of behavioral psychotherapy: theory and practice. *Am. J. Psychiatry,* **133,** 253–261

Skinner, B. F. (1974). *About Behaviourism.* (London: Jonathan Cape)

Chapter 11

COGNITIVE RESTRUCTURING

I. RATIONAL EMOTIVE THERAPY

Rational emotive therapy (RET) a technique developed by Albert Ellis, emphasizes the rational core of man and the control of emotion through the thought process. It is based on the assumption that thought and emotion interact closely, and that for any emotion to be sustained it must be reinforced by the thought process. Therefore, to control emotion in a client one should explore his thought processes and show him how certain thoughts are illogical and unrealistic and then how they can become less so.

Ellis proposed that our cognitive understanding of events, when mistaken, can lead us to maladaptive behaviour. These mistaken beliefs or self-statements are learned early in life. People make such irrational statements as, 'I must never make a mistake; if I did, it would be horrible', or 'I should always act pleasant. I would destroy other people by being angry at them'. Rational emotive therapy, is based on the premise that through extensive talking with clients the therapist can lead them to see the irrational nature of their self-statements and bring them to a more appropriate way of viewing the world.

APPLICATION

Concentrating primarily on the specific illogical thoughts disturbing the client, the therapist must teach him or her to rethink these internalized sentences. He must also work on a number of general irrational ideas which many people hold, to be sure the patient does not substitute one of these other problems for this original one. There are a number of these general illogical ideas which Ellis believed should be worked through with

127

any client (1958). A few of these ideas are, (1) Certain acts are completely wrong and wicked, and one must be punished for them, (2) an adult must be loved and approved by everyone for everything he or she does, and (3) it is easier to avoid life's difficulties and responsibilities than to face them. The therapist must act as a 'counterpropagandist', contradicting these self-defeating thoughts as much as possible. In whatever way he can, the rational therapist should direct the patient to act in a manner contradictory to his or her illogical thoughts. If the patient is afraid to speak to women, the therapist must direct him to speak to some women, and thus show him that the terrible thoughts he has had about what would happen did not come true.

The therapy usually includes (but is not limited to) the following procedural steps:

(1) verbal persuasion aimed at convincing the client of the philosophical tenets of RET
(2) identification of irrational thoughts through client self-monitoring and therapist's feedback
(3) the therapist directly challenges irrational ideas, and models rational reinterpretation of disturbing events
(4) repeated cognitive rehearsal aimed at substituting rational self-statement for previously irrational interpretation
(5) behavioural tasks designed to develop rational reactions.

Ellis certainly did not reject the use of other techniques, especially if the client was particularly upset when he first came to therapy. Expressive techniques such as role playing and free association can aid greatly. He did warn, however, that these other techniques are not doing the real work of therapy, which is dissuading the client from her illogical thoughts, and aiding her to think in a more rational fashion. Ellis also made the point that this form of therapy is limited in the type of client that it can aid. Some people are not intelligent enough to understand the rational thought process, others are too emotionally upset to follow logical procedures, while still others are too rigid in their illogical thought processes to gain anything from this therapy.

EVALUATION

In his review of the clinical and personality hypotheses that provide the basis for the RET system of therapy, Ellis (1977) concluded that the research support for RET is 'immense indeed, almost awesome'.

Several studies provide support for the general notion that thoughts or self-statements can elicit emotional arousal (e.g. May, 1977; Rimm and Litvak, 1969). However, a recent study by Rogers and Craighead (1977) calls into question the pivotal assumption behind RET that specific negative self-statements mediate emotional states. In this study the subject cognitively rehearsed self-referent statements while physiological responses were monitored. There were no differences between either positive or negative self-statements and neutral self-statements on any physiological response (heart rate, skin conductance and finger pulse volume). The only significant finding was that negative self-statements of moderate discrepancy generated greater arousal than moderately discrepant but positive self-statements. Rogers and Craighead concluded that the relationship between cognitions and emotional arousal is more complex than that proposed by Ellis. Further evidence indicating the greater complexity of the interaction between thoughts and feelings than that assumed by Ellis comes from LaPointe and Harrell's (1978) study of correlational relationships between specific cognitions and particular affective states. Surprisingly few significant correlations were found. Goldfried and Davison (1976), in favour of Ellis, report that two of Ellis's notions are especially characteristic of neurotic clients – that 'everybody must love me' and 'I must be perfect in everything I do'. However, these statements of belief are too global and imprecise. For example, few clients believe that literally 'everybody must love me'. Rather, this means that the client wishes that a few highly significant people love him or her.

In sum, these studies do not provide adequate information on which to reach firm conclusions about the efficacy of RET as a treatment method. Evidence on the long-term efficacy of RET is lacking. Encouragingly, in most studies, the evidence suggests that RET is more effective than no-treatment or placebo influences on some measures. However, it is not possible to conclude that RET is superior to alternative treatment methods such as systematic desensitization, prolonged exposure or behavioural rehearsal.

Ellis (1977) argued that RET has been misinterpreted as a treatment approach that is restricted to cognitive restructuring by means of verbal persuasion and logical analysis. He asserts that RET, among other procedures, includes the use of all behaviour therapy techniques, encounter group exercises, Gestalt methods, psychodrama procedures and unconditional acceptance of the client. This turns it into something of a hotch potch.

II. SELF-INSTRUCTIONAL TRAINING

A second form of cognitive restructuring is self-instructional training (SIT), developed by Meichenbaum (1977). The rationale for this approach derives from two main sources: (1) Ellis's (1970) RET and its emphasis on irrational self-talk as the cause of emotional disturbance, and (2) the developmental sequence according to which children develop internal speech and verbal–symbolic control over their behaviour (Luria, 1961). According to this analysis children's behaviour is first regulated by the instructions of other people; subsequently they acquire control over their own behaviour, through the use of overt self-instructions which they ultimately internalize as covert self-instructions. SIT involves the following steps:

(1) training the client to identify and become aware of maladaptive thoughts (self-statements)
(2) the therapist models appropriate behaviour while verbalizing effective action strategies; these verbalizations include an appraisal of task requirements, self-instructions that guide graded performance, self-statements that stress personal adequacy and counteract worry over failure, and covert self-reinforcement for successful performance
(3) the client then performs the target behaviour while verbalizing aloud the appropriate self-instructions, and later by covertly rehearsing them. Therapist feedback during this phase assists in ensuring that constructive problem-solving self-talk replaces previously anxiety-inducing cognitions associated with that behaviour.

SIT was derived, in part, from Ellis's RET and there are important similarities, as well as some conceptual and procedural differences.

Where Ellis tends to focus on his set of 'core irrational ideas', Meichenbaum has seemed to be more interested in idiosyncratic thought patterns. The latter has also devoted more attention to the role of graduated practice in his cognitive training package. In addition, self-instructional training presents a somewhat more heterogeneous package which contains elements of desensitization, modelling, and behaviour rehearsal. Of particular note is the fact that this approach emphasizes practical coping skills for dealing with problematic situations. While the major emphasis of RET is the destruction of maladaptive beliefs, self-instructional training supplants this with a constructive phase of skills development. Where RET highlights the rationality of a thought – believing that rationality is synonymous with adaptiveness – self-instructional training places more emphasis on its adaptiveness. Thus, while RET deposits differences in the thoughts of normal and distressed persons, a self-instructional therapist would place more emphasis on an individual's methods of coping with those thoughts. In other words, it is not the content or incidence of irrational beliefs that differentiates normal and distressed persons – it is their learned means of coping with these beliefs.

Another procedural difference is that, contrary to Ellis's (1970) style of direct confrontation of clients' irrational ideas, Meichenbaum (1977) adopts a Socratic approach in which therapy is structured so that clients discover for themselves the inaccuracies and distortions in their thinking. The client is helped to identify and alter automatic thoughts through a more gentle and strategic progression of therapeutic intervention.

III. BECK'S COGNITIVE THERAPY

A third approach to cognitive restructuring is Beck's (1976) 'cognitive therapy'. Beck (1963) developed this cognitive approach to the under-standing and treatment of clinical disorders, particularly depression, independently of Ellis's RET. There is considerable overlap among these cognitive restructuring procedures. As in RET and self-instructional training, the ultimate goal of cognitive therapy is the development of adaptive thought patterns. Cognitive therapy includes the following basic phases:

(1) clients become aware of their thoughts
(2) they learn to identify inaccurate or distorted thoughts
(3) these inaccurate thoughts are replaced by accurate, more objective cognitions, and
(4) the therapist provides feedback and reinforcement for cognitive and behavioural change.

The specific procedures used to accomplish these therapeutic objectives are described in a treatment manual (Beck, Rush, Shaw and Emery, 1977). They are both behavioural and cognitive in nature. The former include the prescription of an explicit activity schedule, graded tasks aimed at providing mastery and success experiences and various homework assignments. The latter include several techniques of which 'distancing' and 'decentering' are examples. Distancing is the ability to view one's thoughts more objectively, to draw a distinction between 'I believe' (an opinion that is open to disconfirmation) and 'I know' (an 'irrefutable' fact). Teaching these clients to separate themselves from vicariously experiencing the adversities of others is known as decentering. For example, an agoraphobic woman, hearing that a friend of her neighbour died of a heart attack, becomes anxious over the same thing happening to her family.

Further reading

Ellis, A. (1958). Rational Psychotherapy. *J. Gen. Psychol.*, **59**, 35–49
Ellis, A. and Harper, R. (1975). *A New Guide to Rational Living*. (Hollywood: Wilshire Book Co.)

Section IV
HUMANISTIC APPROACHES

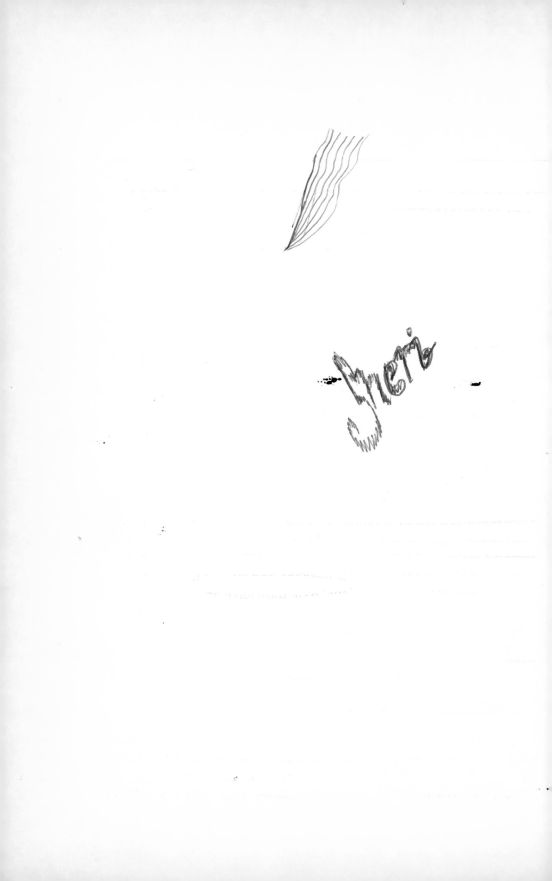

Chapter 12

HUMANISTIC–EXISTENTIAL THERAPIES – AN OVERVIEW

The category of therapies designated as 'existential–humanistic' refers to a number of loosely related approaches that have some elements in common. Humanistic psychology arose in the 1950s largely as a reaction to the prevailing traditions of behaviourism and psychoanalysis. It aimed to evolve a psychology which dealt adequately with people as human beings, not as objects or machines. It emphasizes that people are capable of self-awareness, that they have the power to choose and to direct their own actions, that they are guided by purpose and meaning, and they are capable of responsibility and concern for others. The American Association for Humanistic Psychology offers its field of interest as follows:

> Humanistic psychology is primarily an orientation toward the whole of psychology rather than a distinct area or school. It stands for the respect for the work of persons, respect for differences of approach, open-mindedness as to acceptable methods, and interest in exploration of new aspects of human behaviour. As a 'third force' in contemporary psychology, it is concerned with topics having little place in existing theories and systems: e.g. love, creativity, self, growth, organism, basic need-gratification, self-actualization, higher values, being, becoming, spontaneity, play, humor, affection, naturalness, warmth, ego-transcendence, objectivity, autonomy, responsibility, meaning, fair-play, transcendental experience, peak experience, courage and related concepts. (AAHP, 1962, p. 2)

The humanistic psychotherapies are not bound by common techniques nor are they a unified school of psychotherapy. Rather they represent an orientation to understanding human beings. All are outgrowths of similar philosophical views of the nature of man. Thus, certain similar threads,

135

interwoven in different ways, continue throughout the fabric of these different humanistic therapies.

Therapists who use these therapies stress self-actualization as the basis for psychological growth. They emphasize subjective and immediate experience, awareness and the concept of free choice. They believe that we choose to behave as we do and to perceive things as we do, and therefore we are personally responsible for our actions and perceptions. They focus on the whole person rather than on specific psychological processes. Humanistic therapists are concerned with the uniqueness of each individual, and they focus on the person's natural tendency toward growth and self-actualization. The humanistic therapist does not interpret the client's behaviour (as would a psychoanalyst) or try to modify it (as would a behaviour therapist). The goal of the humanistic therapist is to facilitate exploration of the individual's own thoughts and feelings and to assist the individual in arriving at his or her own solutions. This approach will become clearer as we look at some of the more widely used existential–humanistic therapies. The focus on subjective awareness implies an existential perspective, for one particular aspect of conscious experience is an awareness of being intrinsically involved in the process of existence. For example, we are aware of the passage of time and that we are part of this, with old age and eventual death approaching inexorably. We are aware of being 'inside' ourselves and separate from other people and the world around.

So, humanistic psychologists are concerned with the content of conscious awareness – the way people experience, and make sense of their world. They are also interested in helping people to use their awareness to take more responsibility for who they are and what they do and to create new and more satisfying ways of feeling, acting and relating to other people. The goal is self-actualization – helping people to develop and explore their potential as individuals.

Many of the topics which interest humanistic psychologists, cannot be simulated in a laboratory experiment divorced from real life. Investigations of conscious awareness, through introspection and interviews, produce qualitative material which cannot be quantified without the loss of essential human aspects. There is relatively little use made, therefore, of controlled laboratory experiments and statistical analysis, or explanations in terms of laws and principles (cf behaviourism). Humanistic psychologists do not believe in the possibility of an ultimate 'science of behaviour' in which explanation of specific actions can be made by reference to a common set of laws and variables applying to all people. Much of significance in human experience will remain ineffable (i.e.

impossible to describe). People are not fixed entities. Because of their capacity to be aware of themselves and to initiate change, they have the ability to modify and create the kind of person they can be. Change is continuous, hence explanations in terms of past events (e.g. Freudian) are insufficient.

The term humanistic should not be confused with the word humane, which means kindly, or caring for others. The humanistic view sees man as being special, in the sense that we are more than just highly developed animals. Therefore, humanistic therapists place great value on relating to the client in a very human and sensitive way; they do not present themselves as an imperious God or a non-feeling manipulator. Of course, successful therapists of every school relate to clients in a human way, but existential–humanistic therapists place this concept as a mandatory *modus vivendi* of the therapy context.

The underlying philosophy that permeates these therapies is that of phenomenology, which as Wylie (1961) succinctly states, is the study of direct awareness. Operated within the ambit of humanistic therapy, it implies this: rather than analysing the person from the standpoint of an external observer (as, for example, when you describe someone as an 'introvert' or a 'delinquent'), the humanistic psychologist tries to work from the perspective or standpoint of the person themselves. In other words, the focus is on subjective awareness, how a person experiences their own world and self. This is the phenomenological approach. This phenomenological perspective is encapsulated in the well known quotation from *'To Kill a Mockingbird'* (Lee Harper):

You never really understand a person until you consider things from his point of view – until you climb into his skin and walk around in it.

This is, of course, an impossible counsel of perfection; but as we will emphasize shortly, one of the major characteristics regarded as a vital possession in humanistic therapists, particularly those practising the client-centred approach, is empathy. The emphasis is on understanding, particularly the client's feelings. The therapist must understand and be 'in touch' with the client's feelings, since it is primarily these feelings that he works to redirect.

The phenomenological approach in psychology then is a perspective which attempts to understand man through the impressions of the perceiving subject, and not through the eyes of an observer of the subject. It seeks to understand how the individual views himself; how his needs, feelings, values, beliefs and unique perception of his environment influence him to behave as he does. Behaviour is a function of the personal meanings attached to an individual's perception of past and con-temporaneous experiences. We cannot change events but we can change our perceptions and interpretations of them. Therapy does just this; it does not 'remove' a problem but enables the client to perceive himself in a new way and cope more effectively.

Perception is the central concept in phenomenology and refers to the processes of selecting, organizing and interpreting material into a coherent construction of the psychological environment. This environ-ment has variously been termed the 'perceptual field', the 'psychological field', the 'phenomenal field' or 'life space'. But terminology apart, we are concerned with personal meanings that exist for any person at any instant and which determine his behaviour. Behaviour for a phenomeno-logist can only be understood from the point of view of the behaving individual. Reality exists not in the event itself but in the unique perception of the event. Perceptions are selective, and are often quite erroneous as a result of the distortions engendered by motives, goals, attitudes and defence mechanisms (Bruner and Goodman, 1947). The old adage 'seeing is believing' is perhaps closer to the truth when reversed as 'Believing is seeing'.

A tenet of both cognitive psychology and phenomenology, then, is that behaviour is the result of the individual's perception of the situation, as it appears to him at the moment. Perception is other than what is physically out there. Yet what is perceived is 'reality' to the perceiver, the only reality by which he can guide his behaviour. The phenomenological approach to behaviour, into which the self-concept has become cemented as a major theme, interprets behaviour in terms of the phenomenal field of the subject, and not in terms of analytical categories imposed by an observer. That is to say that behaviour can best be understood as growing out of the individual.

It makes a great deal of difference to how you perceive your work situation if you see yourself as a successful or unsuccessful employee, boss or apprentice. Depending on the pupil's self-concept an examination can be viewed as a challenge or something to avoid, and the front row of the class-room can be perceived as under the eye of the teacher or the best place for hearing and seeing him. This selective perception also enhances existing perceptions, and makes them more difficult to change. The person who considers himself inept at home decorating is likely to avoid such work or by developing high levels of anxiety when doing it, produce inadequate results on a task he believes himself incapable of doing anyway. All this validates his initial hypothesis about himself. It would seem that the very act of initiating a negative perception almost ensures that subsequent behaviour will produce evidence to support the perception. This has been called the 'boomerang effect', a self-fulfilling prophecy. Happily this prophecy works equally well with positive self-attitudes, so that supportive evidence tends to augment and nourish favourable self-concepts.

An optimistic view of people is promoted, as too the assumption that patients inherently improve through their own effort with some guidance from the therapist. In contrast to dynamic therapies, it is perhaps best to think of the process of humanistic psychotherapies as principally a releasing process rather than a reconstruction.

Further reading

Ornstein, R. E. (1977). *Psychology of Consciousness*. (New York: Harcourt Brace Jovanovich)

Spiegelberg, H. (1972). *Phenomenology in Psychology and Psychiatry*. (Evanston, Ill: Northwestern University Press)

Shaffer, J. (1978). *Humanistic Psychology*. (Englewood Cliffs: Prentice Hall)

Chapter 13

THE EXISTENTIAL APPROACH

THEORY

This approach was a philosophical fore-runner in Europe of what became in America the Humanist movement, as exemplified by Rogers' (1961) early book '*On Becoming a Person*'. The existentialists were a combined response to three issues:

Industrialization and alienation

Such early sociologists as Durkheim, Marx and Weber were preoccupied with the declining sense of community in Western Europe, the emergence of mass culture, and the dehumanization that seemed to accompany the growth of the modern industrial State. Science appeared to have made life actually more difficult by presenting the image of a universe without any purpose. With the evolution of the modern technocracy, man has been alienated from his land, his community, his family and his religion. But most significantly, according to the existentialists, man has become alienated from himself. People have become identified with their social functions (e.g. their jobs, their roles), and the remainder of their being drops below the surface of consciousness; this loss of self and self-consciousness produces free-floating anxiety and despair. Thus, the existentialists and the sociologists agreed that the Industrial Revolution had produced widespread anomie; however, the existentialists rejected the sociological explanation of the cause of anomie, that individual states of consciousness are caused by forces outside the person.

Hegelian philosophy

The second source of modern existentialist thought was a vehement and somewhat irrational reaction against the implications of Hegelian philosophy, which stressed that what is highest in the realm of being is highest in the realm of abstraction; the universal is more important than the particular, the abstract is more valuable than the concrete. The major thrust of existentialism is to reverse this Hegelian scale of values and to insist on the significance of the concrete, particular and unique individual.

Freudian psychoanalysis

The third root of modern existentialism comes from psychiatry in the form of a critique of Freud and psychoanalysis. The early existentialist psychiatrists (e.g. Binswanger) found several implications of psycho-analysis objectionable. First, in his preoccupation with biological drives, Freud suggested that a major problem in life is man's relationship to his own body. The existentialists point out that one's relationships with oneself and with others are equally problematical. Second, Freud was an advocate of scientism and technical reason. According to the existent-ialists, however, to analyse men in terms of technical reason leads precisely to the fragmentation that psychoanalysis was trying to cure. In this sense they regard Freud as an agent of the technocracy, as part of the problem rather than the cure. Third, psychoanalysis imposes interpret-ations on people; however, a responsible therapist must ask himself if he is seeing a patient as he really is, or if he is projecting his theories onto the patient.

Although existentialism emerged in its present form as a protest movement, it has made substantive and methodological contributions to the personological tradition. The substantive contribution stems originally from Kierkegaard (1954) who thought the anomie found in modern society was caused by man's inability to find a purpose for his existence. The central problem in existentialism is the meaning of life – and religion has historically supplied this meaning. Kierkegaard, however, was writing out of a world in which God was dying and sought some basis on which the essential worth of the individual could be re-established. Thus, the point of existentialism is not to despair over a Godless world. Rather the movement recasts the problem of meaning in terms of the individual: each person must question radically the purpose of his life and see what answers emerge. The substantive contributions of Kierkegaard and Nietzsche can be summarized as follows. They argue that contemporary man feels alienated from society and himself. This alienation results from the failure of the Judeo–Christian tradition in industrial society; modern science in particular has undermined religion. As a result we are confronted with the problem of meaning, and the major task in life is to deal with this problem in a responsible way.

The existentialist's primary concern is how to describe man as emerging and becoming in his entirety, not as a collection of Behaviourist mechanisms or Freudian dynamics. If one sees man only as such a collection, one has then lost sight of the basic fact of that individual's existence. Existential therapy is an attempt to do away with the division of subject and object so dominant in Western thought. Since the Renaissance, Western thought has concentrated on the essence or basic principles and laws of various problems such as human behaviour. To understand reality it has attempted to separate it into discrete parts. The totality of existence was often ignored.

Dasein

'Being in the world' or 'dasein' is the fundamental concept and password of existentialism. As Binswanger (1955) put it:

> the existential analyst will always stand on the same level with his patients, namely on the level of their common reality (Dasein). Consequently he will not turn the patient into an object in contrast to himself as a subject but will regard him as a partner in human reality (Dasein). He will regard the relationship as a meeting on what Martin Buber has called the 'abyss of human reality' . . . and will denote it not only as self but also as 'Being with' in personal intercourse and as 'Being together' or love. And in an existential sense the condition which Freud has taught us to call transference is also a mode of the meeting (p. 304).

The phenomenological analysis of everyday social life provides a number of interesting insights into human affairs. Beginning with Heidegger (1949), the existentialists distinguish between a form of existence that characterizes non-human objects (Vorhandensein) and one that is peculiar to human beings (Dasein). The difference is that objects (e.g. ships, stones, inkwells) are formed or created by forces outside themselves; man, however, must make himself. Man becomes what he makes of himself and nothing more. Heidegger's *Being and Time* is a phenomenological analysis of the structure of Dasein; his book strongly influenced the psychiatrist Ludwig Binswanger, whose approach is called Dasein-analyse. *Dasein* means 'to be there' and is usually translated as 'existence'. This 'being' is in relation to the entire surrounding world, not just one or two aspects or specific objects of it. The concept of an individual surrounded in a world is very important in the existential therapist's understanding of his clients. Using the concept of being-in-the-world, Binswanger for example, showed that there were character-istic ways of living and moving within one's space, which became important in his method of dream analysis. Also implied by the concept of Dasein is that one is aware of this existence and because of this awareness is able to make choices and decisions about one's life. Binswanger distin-guished three modes of Dasein, three ways of 'being in the world'. The first is called *Umwelt*, a natural manner of living if one lacks self-aware-ness. Umwelt refers to man's physiological desires. 'It is the world of natural law and natural cycles, of sleep and awakeness, of being born and dying, desire and relief, the world of finiteness and biological deter-minism, the 'thrown world' to which each of us must in some way adjust' (May, 1958, p. 61).

The existentialist school of psychiatry understands that biological reality sets fixed limits for us, yet it maintains that there is more to us than physiology. The second mode of Dasein is called the *Mitwelt*, the world of being with other people. The Mitwelt is the world of interpersonal relations; there are four existential modes in the Mitwelt. The first is called the dual mode; here relationships are characterized by warmth, trust, and personal intimacy – the sociological concept of community is an example of the dual mode of the Mitwelt. The dual mode is an existential ideal: it is the desired form of interpersonal relations. The second way of living in the Mitwelt is called the plural mode; this refers to formal inter-actions (e.g. lectures, wedding ceremonies) and to relationships characterized by competition and rivalry. The singular mode is a third way of being in the Mitwelt; the singular mode refers to all forms of narcissistic, self-orientated social behaviour – masturbation and suicide are examples of the singular mode. Finally, the fourth existential mode of Mitwelt is called anonymous. People adopt the anonymous mode when they want to avoid responsibility for their own lives; according to Binswanger, the anonymous mode is typical of soldiers and bureaucrats.

The third and final way of being in Dasein is called the *Eigenwelt*, or own world and refers to self-related, self-aware, self-actualizing ways of being. Eigenwelt is a way of understanding what things in the world mean explicitly for oneself and one's development.

Umwelt is defined almost entirely in terms of adjustment, adaptation, and accommodation – one adjusts to cold weather, hunger and dirty air. Eigenwelt is a world made up almost exclusively of assimilation – the meaning of flowers, trees, or other people is grasped in terms of what they mean for oneself. Mitwelt, however, synthesizes Umwelt and Eigenwelt: it is a mode of being that contains a balance between adjustment and assimilation. The term that best characterizes Mitwelt is relationship. If I force others to adjust to me, to adapt themselves to my desires and expectations, I treat them as objects and dehumanize them; on the other hand, if I constantly adjust to the expectations of others, I dehumanize myself. A relationship is the ideal, dual mode of the Mitwelt and is called an encounter – a relationship with another in which both participants are open to the possibilities of mutual influences and change. As May (1958, p. 38) observes, an ' . . . encounter with the being of another person has the power to shake one profoundly and may potentially be very anxiety-arousing. It may also be joy-creating. In either case, it has the power to grasp and move one deeply'. Although each mode of Dasein refers to a distinctive style of being, it is important to remember that we live in all three modes simultaneously. Moreover, something is lost from our lives if we emphasize one mode of being to the exclusion of the others. Lives oriented primarily to pleasure, to social interaction, or self-realization are immature.

It was mentioned earlier that people differ from objects primarily in that people define or create themselves. People are characterized by what Binswanger called world-openness, or the capacity for transcendence. This is related to one of the most important issues in existentialist thought: antideterminism. Man can achieve transcendence (and escape the bonds of determinism) in two ways. He can free himself from the constraints of his own thought processes – psychic reality – by becoming self-conscious about them; i.e. he can transcend psychic reality by making his mental processes the objects of psychological study. Man can free himself from physical reality through his capacity for world-openness, i.e. through his ability to restructure reality in his own terms.

Angst

People generally tend to avoid facing the problem of meaning; when they do, however, they tend to experience Angst, an emotion imperfectly translated by the words anxiety and dread. Angst is a subjective state in which a person is intensely aware of the possibility of non-being, of the fact that he can be destroyed. In his classic analysis of anxiety, Kierkegaard argued that people are never motivated by pleasure, happiness or sex; they are motivated by dread, by anxiety over the possibility of non-being.

The Angst that resuls from the apparent purposelessness of human existence is more than most people can bear. Therefore, according to Kierkegaard and Nietzsche, most people choose not to ask about the meaning of their lives, and their resulting loss of self-awareness can be described as self-deception. Thus, most people are self-deceived, there are neurotic consequences that flow from this self-deception, and the cure is self-knowledge. The same theme is found in Heidegger who argued that the most authentic or 'human' mode of Being was to be self-reflective. Those who are self-deceived are alienated from themselves; those who are self-aware are authentic.

Roles

For George Herbert Mead (1934) the self-concept is defined socially; it is determined by the roles one plays, and reflects how one sees oneself from the perspective of one's family and associates. The existentialists, however, distinguish between the self and the self-concept and define the former in terms of self-consciousness. The self is not the product of one's roles; rather it is the capacity to know that one is playing a role; it is the ability to see oneself in many roles. For the existentialists then, the self-concept in Mead's sense is something to be overcome. To the degree that a person cannot step outside his social roles and see them in perspective, i.e. that one is identified with one's self-concept or social roles, he is self-deceived; he has become an object because he is exogenously (socially) defined; he lives in 'bad faith'.

We each develop a repertoire of roles and our lives come to resemble an extended sequence of stage performances, some of which require profound changes of costume and demeanour. Socialization is, of course, equated with the internalization of these roles. The more intensely one had internalized one's roles, the more one is socialized. Roles often conflict, producing inconsistencies in one's performances from time to time. To avoid anxiety over these inconsistencies, people commonly dissociate or segregate their consciousness as well as their roles. They don't repress awareness of role inconsistencies, because the concept of repression makes no sense from an existentialist perspective, rather they redirect their attention. Thus, most people are sincere as they play their roles because, once again, sincerity is easier to maintain than self-awareness. Sincerity is the psychological state of one who believes his own act.

But a person lives in bad faith if he plays his roles with sincerity and inner identification; one lacks self-awareness and is self-deceived. Human dignity requires role distance, an inner detachment from one's social situation; it requires self-awareness. Thus, for the existentialists, conventional socialization, like the socially defined self-concept, is something to be overcome.

Thus people are alike in that they need meaning, and they respond to the lack of meaning with Angst and self-deception. From an existentialist perspective anxiety and guilt are never undesirable *per se*. Because intellectual honesty inevitably leads to the problem of meaning and an encounter with the absurd, Angst is the first sign of intellectual awakening. Angst may subsequently serve as a stimulus for personal growth. Therefore, psychological health is not defined by an absence of anxiety but rather by using the proper means to deal with it.

Neurosis

The existentialists distinguish between Angst, normal guilt, and neurotic guilt. Angst results from the problem of meaning, guilt on the other hand is a product of one's life-style. Normal guilt arises when a person denies his potentialities or fails to fulfill them. Neurotic guilt arises from a failure to acknowledge normal guilt, from a refusal to deal with it in a responsible way. For the existentialists neurotic and psychotic symptoms are seen as techniques for reducing neurotic guilt. Typically these symptoms have the effect of allowing one to avoid responsibility for his own life.

Neurotic symptoms are always somewhat effective in that they allow a neurotic to preserve his sense of personal worth. According to Rollo May (1958), sickness is precisely the method the neurotic uses to preserve his own being. Because the existentialists feel modern society is dehumanizing, they tend to be sympathetic with their clients. Often a neurotic life-style is the best that a person can manage, given his life circumstances. Moreover, people are changing constantly, and one must continually adapt to the demands of life. Thus happiness now is no guarantee of happiness later; in a real sense, life consists of one crisis of existence after another – as H. L. Mencken said, 'Life is just one damned thing after another'.

Although the existentialists have some sympathy for neurotics, their predominant attitude is actually more ambivalent. In '*The Sickness Unto Death*', Kierkegaard (1954) suggested two general principles, concerning neurosis. First, we never feel anxiety or despair over external objects but always over ourselves, i.e. we don't despair over the loss of a job but over the image we have of ourselves as jobless. Second, what we call neurosis is actually a form of sinfulness. There is a tendency to regard morally deficient people as sick, mentally ill or neurotic. The closer we get to any neurotic, the more we are struck by his perversity and wilful disagreeableness. In Sartre's terms, a neurotic, one who has undergone a 'mental breakdown', is in fact self-deceived; he is a coward who flees from self-awareness and personal responsibility. Nietzsche referred to neurotics as 'pale felons', as would-be villains who do not have the courage of their immoral convictions; they lack sufficient nerve to affirm their existence as great scoundrels and they are content with perpetrating petty crimes on other people – by being late for appointments, forgetting to return items they borrow, being unreasonably moody, etc.

If neurotics are victims of mental disease, then our proper response should be pity and compassion. If, however, neurotics are self-deceived, then our response should be the same as that which we have toward any other form of cowardice. The neurotic must be led firmly, but tactfully, to self-awareness; he must be persuaded to confront as much reality as his courage will bear. If neurotics are self-deceived cowards, then psycho-therapy becomes a moral rather than a medical enterprise.

EXISTENTIAL CRITERIA OF PSYCHOLOGICAL HEALTH

Drawing on all the material presented above, there seem to be five criteria that, from an existentialist perspective, define psychological health. First, as May (1958) observes, neurotics are overconcerned with the Umwelt and underconcerned with the Eigenwelt. Thus the healthy person is one who has established a proper balance among the three modes of Dasein. In particular, psychological health is denoted by the capacity for significant interpersonal relationships: it is the capacity to live in the dual mode of the Mitwelt.

Second, as Allport noted, psychological health requires engagement, a commitment to life and the pursuit of certain personally chosen goals therein. Camus once remarked that the only important philosophical question was whether or not to commit suicide. The fact that a person does not shoot himself means that he has made an affirmation. He then has a responsibility to live up to that affirmation by making a commitment to life. Consequently, we must pursue our goals as vigorously as possible, realizing that they are quite arbitrary but must be pursued nonetheless.

A third criterion of psychological health is the capacity to assume responsibility for one's life. Sartre's refusal to accept the Nobel prize for literature is perhaps an example of this. Sartre claimed that he refused the prize in part because he felt the Nobel committee, in offering it to him, was also offering to forgive him for some of the ideas and actions of his youth. Sartre maintained that his youthful behaviour had seemed valid at the time and, although he had subsequently changed his mind, he would not disavow those earlier actions in the present. He had meant them at the time, they were part of him, and to deny them now would be an evasion.

Thus, the existentialist notion of responsibility is quite stern; it is not a concept for the faint-hearted or the conventionally ambitious.

A fourth criterion of psychological health is a unified or integrated personality. As stated several times in this book, integration is a problem that psychoanalysis ignores. For the existentialists, dissociation (or lack of integration) results from self-deception. The cure for self-deception is self-awareness, the necessary precondition of integration. In direct contrast with the cult of self-expression that seems so prevalent in parts of our society, the existentialists, along with Freud and the ancient Greeks, argue that self-actualization depends on suppression and self-discipline; only those who are willing to be hard on themselves can attain self-awareness.

Finally, psychological health is characterized by self-consciousness, self-awareness and a willingness to be an individual, to affirm one's own existence, to avoid the anonymous mode of Dasein. Because the self-aware individual is capable of transcendence, he is free.

However, psychological health does not mean happiness; it means living with the knowledge that one's being has no ultimate justification or purpose. In 'The Myth of Sisyphus', Camus (1955) develops an inspired metaphor for man's fate. Sisyphus is condemned to spend eternity pushing a huge boulder up a high hill; each time he reaches the top the boulder rolls back down to the underworld. Similarly, each person struggles through life only to die. Yet Sisyphus does have a task to complete. And during those brief moments he spends at the crest of the hill he can enjoy the breeze and his momentary view from the summit. For these reasons, Camus concludes, we must consider Sisyphus content. Life's final lack of meaning can be transcended by a self-conscious affirmation of an otherwise arbitrary goal. Hence, emphasis is upon the spontaneous moment of experience, and a reluctance to pin down this moment into any explanatory scheme. Facing, and confronting, even though it appears an abyss – this is the nucleus of the existential approach.

The therapeutic approach

The existential approach must be carried out in the continuing therapeutic relationship. The existentialist therapist will not explain or avoid the anxiety which is to take away from the moment; he only indicates, and shares. Practically speaking, this allows the existential therapist to be much more open in his response to the client, pushing the patient towards immediacy and away from the false generalization or categories.

But if the anxiety arises, not from the danger of becoming aware of repressed and invisible wishes, but simply from being unable to face what is there already, then the only help is with facing the horror directly. In Binswanger's well-known case, that of Ellen West, the client had been helped existentially even though the choice she was able to make – by virtue of finding her being-in-the-world – was suicide. Existentialism's concern for shared experience, brings it into line with many of the transcendent approaches, particularly those which draw on the Oriental tradition. It influenced the humanist psychology movement, and the Gestalt approach, with its premium on immediacy. No preconceived theory is used to understand the client's past life. Each individual client is seen as a completely unique individual with a unique background that plays an important role in his or her present being. No assumptions are made about the meaning of past incidents. The meaning can only be discovered by working with the patient. The therapist should not direct the client, but rather should be an existential partner to the client, helping him re-establish communication with others and with himself, which has been lost in some way. Therapy should be understood as an encounter between two individuals who optimally treat each other mutually as subjects and not as objects. Both individuals must feel they are participating in this encounter, and most of the work of the therapy is accomplished in the encounter.

Boss (1957) believed that the procedures developed by Freud and employed by psychoanalysts are the best techniques available for therapy. In fact, he believed that Dasein analysts often adhere more strictly to Freud's techniques than many psychoanalysts. The difference again lies in the way the therapist views her relationship with the patient and the interpretations she makes. There is an important difference between the existential view of what Freud described as transference and the psychoanalytic view. The client's feelings about the analyst are accepted simply as feelings about the analyst and not necessarily as emotions connected to important figures from the client's past. By viewing the relationship between analyst and client as simply one between two individuals, existentialists redirect the emphasis of therapy from discovering causation in the past to exploring feelings and relationships in the present. Gaining insight is part of the process, but insight into the present situation.

Even though many existential analysts do follow the same techniques, Rollo May (1958) has pointed out that in existential therapy the techniques follow understanding in importance. The task is to understand the patient, and have him experience his existence as real by whatever method is best for that client. The therapist must be flexible in his or her use of techniques. The aim of the therapy is not to alleviate a symptom or to help the client 'adjust' to society, but rather to have the client discover her own being. If the therapy is successful, the patients experience their existence as real, and become fully aware of this existence so that options and potentials become evident and change is, therefore, seen as possible. The therapy is seen as helping the client carry out these options in life; it influences decision making and helps the client achieve an attitude of commitment in his or her life. This effect of the treatment is especially appropriate given the concept of an existential neurosis in which emotional problems are not the result of repression of drives or pathological object relations, but rather the result of an inability to see life as meaningful.

One of the most influential British existentialists is R. D. Laing, although, like all good existentialists, he resists classification. Laing is true to existentialism by refusing to define a system or allow himself to get pinned down to any particular concept. The flavour of Laing's existentialism is illustrated in the following statements, taken from his book 'The Politics of Experience' (1970): 'No one can begin to think, feel or act now except from the starting point of his or her own alienation', 'Psychotherapy must remain an obstinate attempt of two people to recover the wholeness of being human through the relationship between them', and again 'Existence is a flame which constantly melts and recasts our theories. Existential thinking offers no security, no home for the homeless. It addresses no one except you and me'.

Laing actively implicates the environment – particularly the family – as the alienating agent. Consequently, Laing is not content to merely tolerate madness as a valid form of experience, it becomes rather an act of heroism, a positive virtue, an attack against alienated culture. The real madness is of those in power, from parent to government, the psychotic, socially defined, is potentially freed by his exclusion from society's power and bureaucracy. Medical establishment stands for repression and segregation of the deviant–insane; the antipsychiatry of existentialism stands for rebellious madness, an acceptable behavioural response to the conventional 'madness' of everyday society, like the BBC's 'Goon Show' as a sane programme in an insane world. Laing has also called attention to the pernicious labelling and social objectification of the psychotic. Laingians have tended to consider neurosis or psychosis as wholly a matter of social alienation – instead of a self-alienation which may begin in a setting of social alienation but then takes on a course of its own for which the individual himself is responsible.

EVALUATION

Looking first at the short-comings, existentialist writers express themselves in terms of the most inconsistent and ambiguous language in philosophy or psychology. This undisciplined language reflects to some degree the literary origins of the movement, but for the most part it is intentional and deliberate, a self-conscious repudiation of technical reason and scientific discourse. Although their hostility to scientism is understandable, their murky language is a poor instrument of intellectual reform.

Second, the level of self-awareness required to live in good faith is itself unrealistic. According to Sartre, then, self-deception is built into the nature of consciousness. The most we can accomplish with diligent self-scrutiny is to narrow the gap between the unknowable free self and the self known by introspection. Self-awareness is an unattainable goal.

A third problem with existentialism is that the movement is essentially leaderless. This chapter seriously misrepresents the organization and structure of existentialism, which in fact is an unstructured gathering of loosely related ideas and theoretical positions.

Fourthly, Laing may have performed a major disservice to the treatment of schizophrenia. Schizophrenia is a real disorder within the individual – one that can have a biological basis, too, as well as an environmental one. Laingian ideas are virtually inapplicable to the great majority of actual psychotics, whose desperate social and personal position would never permit even the beginning of existential treatment.

Finally, along with Freud, the existentialists present us with a tragic view of life, a view that seems neither sustained nor understood by the other contributors to the personological tradition. For the existentialists, as for Freud, happiness is not possible; indeed, there is something a bit odd about those who pursue it. Life is pointless, death a certainty, and within those two unassailable realities one must find a meaning for oneself. The emphasis is on action despite the fact that such action is inevitably futile. However, it is an important antidote to the experimental methodology to which American psychology seems wedded.

Existential therapy will not remove the feelings of estrangement, since its essentially individualistic structure only further cuts a person off from the dimension of real social causes and remedies that apply to alienation in all its forms. By simply cultivating the experience and denying recourse to interpretative explanations, the client is left wallowing in immediate subjectivity. Explanation does permit an appreciation and understanding of current experience as a continuation of old forms of behaviour. The existential approach is basically myopic, unable to see a world of form and depth.

The advantage of existentialism is that the intensification of awareness leads the individual to question all ready-made explanations, and makes possible a new leap. And by minimizing explanation, it minimizes the chance for rationalization (e.g. 'I'm sick because my parents made me so') and thus promotes acceptance of responsibility for one's life.

The existential approach is the most radical of all the therapeutic strategies. It posits pure consciousness as the object of therapeutic attention. The existential approach thrusts us into our very being and removes explanatory support (It's only your nerves') and cannot be other than a radical method if seriously applied. By removing explanatory props, the existential puts us face to face with experience and distress – that is to say, with the demonic; to take full responsibility for it, such being the condition of freedom.

The existential attitude mainly defines a line of approach to emotional disorder, and is not in itself a complete therapy. Nonetheless, the approach itself may be a useful way of homing in on neurotic distress wherever the neurosis is combined with acute feeling of alienation from the world. Generally speaking, such a condition is felt by people of rather heightened self-awareness who have lost faith in traditional reassurances, whether these be of reason or of faith.

Further Reading

Boss, M. (1963). *Psychoanalysis and Daseinanalysis*. (New York: Basic Books)

Laing, R. D. (1960). *The Divided Self*. (London: Tavistock)

May, R. (1958). Contributions of existential psychotherapy. In May, R., Angel, E. and Ellenberger, H. F. (eds.) *Existence: A New Dimension in Psychiatry and Psychology*. (New York: Basic Books)

Chapter 14

ROGERS' CLIENT-CENTRED THERAPY

INTRODUCTION

The growth of Rogerian psychotherapy has been one of the more important modern developments in the field of psychotherapy. Phenomenology, with the perceived self-concept as its core, was appropriated by Rogers to underpin his developing client-centred approach to psychotherapy. He was able to describe therapeutic change in terms of a perceptual frame of reference.

Carl Rogers first wrote about his theory in 1942. His early views focused on recognizing and clarifying the client's expressed feelings. At that time the technique was called *non-directive therapy*, because a basic rule was that the therapist should adopt a passive role and only echo the client's own words, never direct the conversation. The purpose of restating clients' feelings was to facilitate the appropriate expression of feelings, to help persons understand how they felt, and to help them use feelings as a basis for action. But gradually, Rogers came to believe that the therapist should be more active, for instance, by responding to subtle emotional cues given by the client rather than merely reflecting what the client says. In 1951, Rogers renamed his approach *Client-Centred Therapy*. In choosing the name 'client-centred', Rogers kept the idea that change and growth comes from within the client, while dropping the idea of a passive therapist, which 'non-directive' clearly implied.

The implication of these terms is that the client has within him the ability and motivation to improve himself, and that the therapist's role is primarily one of facilitating that improvement. The theory is 'humanistic' and hence fits in our everyday language system, which is marked by terms like 'free-will', choice and personal responsibility. Such an approach to human behaviour generally leads to an emphasis on the

153

'self' and on the characteristics of the self concept. In addition, the approach has a flavour of observation rather than intervention. Instead of using experimental phrasing such as 'If I do this to him, then . . .', Rogers thinks this way:

> If certain conditions exist . . . , then a process will occur . . . If this process . . . occurs, then certain personality and behavioural changes . . . will occur. (1959, p. 212)

During the decades since the publication of *Client-Centred Therapy* (Rogers, 1951), Rogers and his co-workers have refined and added to the system. They have incorporated the idea of the self-concept into the theory, and have extended treatment to schizophrenics (Rogers, Gendlin, Kiesler, and Truax, 1967) and to groups (Rogers, 1970). Rogerians also have been actively researching their techniques (Truax and Mitchell, 1971) as well as working out quantitative ways to analyse client-centred therapy (Carkhuff, 1969).

Client-centred therapy is based on the assumption that the client is the best expert on him or herself, and that, given a fair chance, most people can work out the solutions to their own problems. The task of the therapist is to facilitate this progress – not to ask probing questions or to make interpretations or to suggest courses of action. In fact, Rogers prefers the term 'facilitator' to 'therapist'.

THE THEORY

Rogers differs in two ways from most psychotherapists. Firstly, he is hardly influenced by Freud and secondly his academic background leads him to be concerned with scientific standards and assessment of results. Rogers views man's nature as essentially positive, moving towards maturity, socialization and self-actualization. He contends that Freud has presented us with a picture of man who at heart is irrational, unsocialized and destructive of self and others. Rogers accepts that a person may at times function like this, but at such times he is neurotic and not functioning as a full human being. When man is functioning freely, he is open to experience and free to act in a positive, trustworthy and constructive manner:

> One of the most refreshing and invigorating parts of my experience is to work with such individuals and to discover the strongly positive directional tendencies which exist in them, as in all of us at the deepest levels. (Rogers, 1961, p. 27.)

He rejects original sin as a puritanical nonsense indicating Freudian therapy as the major representative of this melancholic perspective of a world of helplessness and hopelessness. Rogers plumbs the depth of man to find there a positive force:

> the innermost core of a man's nature, the deepest layers of his personality, the base of his 'animal nature' is positive in nature – is basically socialized, forward-moving, rational and realistic. (1961, p. 90.)

This is the heart of humanism – rather than attempting to provide insight into repressed memories of the past, the client-centred therapist tries to help clients accept all aspects of themselves in the present. Emotional problems are seen as stemming from a lack of self-knowledge, a denial of certain feelings, and an inability to experience all feelings fully.

However, the Rogerian therapist does not probe beneath the neuroses of the client. Client-centred therapy is based on Rogers' theory of personality, in which the self concept is central. The self concept is defined as a relatively consistent and enduring framework of self-regarding attitudes (Burns, 1979). Disturbed persons are those who find some of their experiences or feelings to be inconsistent with the concept they have of themselves, and so they deny that the feelings apply to them. If the person denies part of his or her own experience, these feelings and experiences cannot be used as a guide for action. For example, one woman in therapy responded to every question about how she felt about a negative event in her life with the comment that she was 'upset'. When asked by the therapist what she meant by 'upset', she said she did not know. Later it was discovered that in her formative years her mother had denied her the implications of any negative feelings. She would say, 'You aren't angry at me, you're upset'. The woman had learned to cut off feelings of anger, depression, jealousy and anxiety. She responded to situations that would normally have elicited such feelings with vague reactions of apprehension and uneasiness. Therapy led her to understand and accept the fact that she has these feelings, and to experience them in appropriate situations. Instead of being confused and disoriented in unpleasant situations, she could respond spontaneously and openly with her feelings. Openly expressing one's feelings is more apt to help resolve the situation causing the negative feelings. For example, people are likely to avoid saying things that make you angry if they know how you feel about such things. Client-centred therapy promotes self-exploration. The therapist tries to develop an environment of acceptance in which clients can take the chance of facing their denied feelings. Clients are encouraged to move to an internal frame of reference in which they decide how worthwhile they are rather than always looking to others for evaluation. Emphasis is placed on the development of a real relationship in therapy rather than on role playing for the therapist.

The self concept is almost indispensable to Rogers when he speaks of human behaviour. It was not always so:

I began my work (1959, p. 200), with the settled notion that the 'self' was a vague, ambiguous, scientifically meaningless term which had gone out of the psychologist's vocabulary with the departure of the introspectionists.

Unfortunately, Rogers' clients insisted on using the term, and slowly he realized that 'in some odd sense . . . (the client's) goal was to become his "real self" ' (1959, p. 200).

Despite the increasing importance of the self concept, its definition remained somewhat vague, and acceptable observable criteria for the construct were unavailable. Attitudes towards self, however, could be studied, and Rogers did so, observing attitudinal changes in therapy. Self attitudes did change in a positive direction, as he predicted, as did attitudes to others.

The self is a concept developed by reflexive thought out of the raw material of stimulus imput. Around the concepts gather evaluative and affective attitudes so that each one becomes good or bad. These evaluative items are internalized from the culture and from others, as well as from self. Rogers' self concept (1951) may be thought of as:

an organized configuration of perceptions of the self . . . It is composed of such elements as the perception of one's characteristics and abilities; the percepts and concepts of self in relation to others and to the environment; the value qualities which are perceived as associated with experiences and objects; and goals and ideals which are perceived as having positive or negative valence (p. 136).

It is the subjective self concept i.e. self perceptions rather than any 'real' self, which is of significance in personality and behaviour. As Snygg and Combs (1949, p. 123) noted the existence of a 'real' self is a philosophical question, since it cannot be observed directly. The self concept becomes the most significant determinant of response to the environment. It governs the perceptions of meanings attributed to the environment. Its sole aim is self-actualization.

Whether learned or inherent, a need for positive regard from others (acceptance, respect, warmth) develops or emerges with the self concept. Rogers leans towards attributing this need to learning. A need for positive self-regard or self-esteem, according to Rogers, is learned through internalization or introjection of being positively regarded by others. Self-regard is derived in large measure from the interpreted regard others have for you (Cooley's looking glass self). This positive regard from others may be conditional or unconditional. When other people with whom the person interacts come to see certain thoughts and behaviours as more or less worthy of regard, the person takes this as conditional positive regard of self; the self becomes selective in thought and behaviour so as to satisfy these 'conditions'.

Two systems have now developed, both of which determine behaviour. The one, based on self-actualization, approaches or avoids depending on whether or not the resulting experience is seen as one which will enhance the person. The other, based on the need for positive regard, approaches or avoids depending on whether or not the resulting experience is seen as one which will meet with approval from significant others (or from the self, when the viewpoint of others has been internalized). Needless to say, the person often encounters situations in which one basic need says 'approach' while the other says 'avoid'. Learning a new skill, for example, often means embarrassment in the early, awkward stages but, when accomplished, adds to the competence of the individual. It is within the conflict of these two basic needs, the need for actualization and the need for positive regard, that the trauma of individual history is enacted. Advance and relapse, adjustment and maladjustment – all can be traced to the working out of an individual solution to this conflict.

As we shall see below, the therapist attempts to convey unconditional positive regard as part of the therapeutic process. To the extent that the need for positive regard dictates choice over the need for actualization, incongruence between self and experience will develop. In Rogers' words, the person:

> has not been true to himself, to his own natural optimistic valuing of experience, but for the sake of preserving the positive regard of others has now come to falsify some of the values he experiences and to perceive them only in terms based upon their value to others (1959, p. 226).

With the incongruence comes vulnerability to threat and anxiety, and defensive distortion of one's experiences. When the incongruence reaches too high a level the person will seek help, or be forced to seek help, from an institution created for such a purpose or from a psychologist, psychiatrist, priest, educational counsellor etc.

An extremely general conceptualization of these two basic needs – for actualization and a need for positive regard – encompasses all significant human behaviour. Since these constructs are so general, they are extremely difficult to find observable criteria for. Rogers does not seem to mind, as long as there is some meaning for a given individual. The therapist's task, after all, is not to intervene but to present a situation of love, honesty and openness. Within such a situation, the best of human motivations can fulfil themselves.

So maladjustment develops if experiences are blocked or distorted, and are prevented from being adequately assimilated into the self concept. Thus, Rogers views maladjustment as a state of incongruence, the most serious source of incongruence being between self and organism. This can arise when a person's self concept is heavily dependent on values and definitions from others that have been internalized. So, incongruence would occur where an individual's self concept heavily stressed love and concern for others, and that person found himself in a situation where as a result of frustration he felt strongly aggressive. These feelings might then be blocked as his self concept could not assimilate the idea that he could hate. Incongruence between self and organism would result. Rogers gives as an example a rejecting mother who cannot admit to herself her feelings of aggression towards her child. She, therefore, perceives his behaviour as bad and deserving punishment. She can then be aggressive towards him without disturbing her self concept of 'good and loving mother' because he is seen as worthy of punishment. The origins of such incongruence between self concept and organismic feelings often lie early in life. Parental affection and 'positive regard' are often conditional on a child disowning his true feelings. If he really does want to smack Mummy then he is a 'bad boy', a person of no merit. Rogers urges instead that parents should indicate to the child that although they understand his feelings he is not allowed to act on them because of the damage or distress such behaviour would cause, rather than express disapproval at the possession of the feelings themselves. The child should thus be encouraged to inhibit the expression of certain feelings rather than disown them. This is a considerable help in avoiding later maladjustment. If parents consistently exhibit unconditional positive regard, the self-regard will likely be unconditional also. This does not mean that a distinction is made between the person and his behaviours. Many religions avow the wisdom of this principle by insisting on the immutable value of the man no matter how heinous his behaviour.

A person with high self-esteem, for example, tends to be well adjusted and more competent both in interpersonal relations and in achievement tasks. An informative introduction to such research can be found in Burns (1979; 1982).

The organism is an integrated whole, to which Rogers attributes, like the organismic theorists, one dynamic drive – that of self-actualization – a basic tendency to 'actualise, maintain and enhance the experiencing organism' (1951, p. 487).

The development of self concept is not just the slow accretion of experiences, conditionings and imposed definitions by others. The self concept is a configuration. Alteration of one aspect can completely alter the nature of the whole. Thus, Rogers is using the term 'self concept' to refer to the way a person sees himself. As he goes on to develop his theory, however, his use of the concept also incorporates the second sense – a process controlling and integrating behaviour. But in Rogers' theory the self concept is not an executive or doer. There is no need for positing such a role. The organism is by nature continually active, seeking its goal of actualization through its constant activity. The self concept thus influences the direction of activity, rather than initiating it and directing it entirely. In this way the self as known and the self as knower are fused. Behaviour is 'the goal directed attempt of the organism to satisfy its needs as experienced in the field as perceived' (1951, p. 491).

In his formulation of the concept of the ideal self, Rogers says that as a result of therapy the perception of the ideal self becomes more realistic, and the self becomes more congruent with the ideal. This suggests that personality disturbance is characterized by an unrealistic self-ideal, and/or incongruence between the self concept and the self-ideal. This formulation has been the basis of some research by the client-centred school (e.g. Butler and Haigh, 1954). Rogers' theory does not emphasize conflict between the self concept and the self-ideal as a source of disturbance, but stresses the conflict between the self concept and organismic experiences as its source. This is in contrast to some other theories in which the self-ideal is a central concept and an important factor in psychological adjustment or maladjustment (e.g. Horney, 1950). He presented the theory to the public in 1951 formulated out of a series of 19 propositions. The first seven refer to the organism and the phenomenological character of the environment, the eighth introduces the concept of self, while the rest form an essay on self psychology. For a full discussion of the self concept, readers are referred to Burns (1979, 1982).

THE TECHNIQUE

Client-centred therapy appears superficially simple, but in practice it requires great skill and is rather more subtle. The therapist begins by explaining the nature of the interviews: the responsibility for working out problems is the client's; he or she is free to leave at any time and to choose whether or not to return; the relationship is a private and confidential one; the client is free to speak of intimate matters without fear of reproof or of having information revealed to others. Once the situation is structured, the clients do most of the talking. Usually they have a good deal to 'get off their chest'. The therapist is an alert but patient listener. When the client stops, as though expecting the therapist to say something, the therapist usually acknowledges and accepts the feelings the client has expressed. For example, if a man has been talking about his nagging wife, the therapist may say, 'You feel that your wife tries to control you'. The object is to clarify the feelings the client has been expressing, not to judge them or to elaborate on them.

During the therapy, the client explores in particular the incongruities in his experience; why he feels one way at one time and then changes, or why he attempts actions which displease him. It is especially important for the client to discover feelings that he has distorted or denied from awareness. Then, the client can come to experience feelings, deep emotional experiences that until then were blocked in some way. He can experience the emotions within the therapeutic situation, even though it may be very disorganizing, because he feels the acceptance and unconditional positive regard of the therapist. He feels safe in presenting even his weakest points to the therapist, because all of what is exposed is met with the same positive regard. Defences are relaxed and he begins to value himself. This leads to a restructuring of his self concept and he accepts feelings that he could not in the past. The client may experience some disorganization of self concept, which then goes through a process of reorganization resulting in a new and more complete self concept. This new self concept is built upon the client's own experiences and not the ideas which others have believed about him or her. Fifth, the client experiences this new self in action. After a period of time, he begins to see his actions are changing along with his new self concept. The client's final responsible act within the therapy is to decide to leave it. The outcome of client-centred therapy is considered in terms of the growth of the individual, and not in terms of the removal of specific symptoms or the social acceptability of the client after therapy. How the client perceives himself or herself in the end is the most important factor in judging the result of this therapy.

Diagnosis is considered not only unnecessary but possibly harmful to the therapeutic interaction, because it may create an image of the therapist as an expert, encouraging the client to form a dependent relationship. It also may give the therapist preconceived ideas about the problems of the client, which must be avoided.

All of this demonstrates a basic phenomenological view of man. In client-centred therapy, the phenomenal field of the individual is all important. It is through perception of oneself that problems arise, and it is through facilitating the change in this perception that the therapist helps the client. The therapist aids the client in gaining 'self-acceptance' and in differentiating the perception of his field, so that the client can better understand, recognize and resolve his problems. The client is able to do this difficult task of restructuring his field because of the special conditions brought about by the therapeutic relationship, which give the client freedom to explore his perceptual field to the fullest, and freedom from any threat to his self concept. The client is considered the only valid source of information about his own phenomenal field. The therapist must believe the client and use the information the client gives him, not any preconceived ideas that the therapist might hold.

The focus is on the client's present feelings, as opposed to past feelings, in an accepting atmosphere where it is all right to feel anything. As therapy progresses, the client becomes more and more aware of feelings that have been denied, and comes to accept those feelings and to incorporate them into the self concept. In short, the client gains a comfortable sense of 'getting it together', which in Rogerian terms means the client is experiencing congruence.

Rogerian therapy sessions are typically held once a week. Generally the clients begin therapy with rather low evaluations of themselves, but in the course of facing up to problems and trying to arrive at solutions, they become more positive. For example, a case may begin with statements such as the following:

'Everything is wrong with me. I feel abnormal. I can't do anything right. I'm inferior. I'm useless.'

By the time of the final interview, the client can be expressing the following attitudes, which contrast strikingly with those of the first interview:

I am taking up a new career of my own choosing. I am really changing. I have always tried to live up to others' standards that were beyond my abilities. I've come to realize that I'm not so bright, but I can get along. I no longer think so much about myself. I'm much more comfortable with people. I'm getting a feeling of success out of my job.

To determine whether this kind of progress is typical, client-centred therapists carefully analyse recorded interviews. When clients' statements are classified and plotted, the course of therapy turns out to be fairly predictable. In the early interviews, people spend a good deal of time talking about their problems, describing symptoms and making negative statements about themselves. During the course of therapy, they make more and more statements that indicate an understanding of their particular problems. By classifying all clients' remarks as either 'problem restatements' or 'statements of understanding and insight', one can see the progressive increase in insight as therapy proceeds. By noting the positive or negative statement made by the client about himself/herself there is also a striking parallel movement from mainly negative to mainly positive self evaluation as therapy progresses.

What do client-centred therapists do to bring about these changes? First of all, they create an atmosphere in which the client feels worthy and significant. The atmosphere develops not as a consequence of technique, but as a result of the therapist's conviction that every person has the capacity to deal constructively with his or her psychological situation. In accepting this viewpoint, therapists cannot merely be passive listeners; if they were, clients might feel that the therapists were not interested in them. The therapists listen intently, and try to show in what they say that they can see things as the client sees them. Rogers emphasizes that the therapist should try to adopt the client's own frame of reference – that is, try to see the problems as the client sees them. To have therapeutic value, the change in the client must be a change of feeling, a change in attitude – not merely a change in intellectual understanding.

Built around the aim of attempting to change the client's view of himself (self concept) the therapy is unashamedly phenomenological as the therapist tries to understand the client from the client's own perspective. Rogers gives a description of the attitude of the counsellor who is trying to assume the client's internal frame of reference:

To be of assistance to you I will put aside myself – the self of ordinary interaction – and enter your world of perception as clearly as I am able. I will become, in a sense, another self for you – an alter ego of your own attitudes and feelings – a safe opportunity for you to discern yourself more truly and deeply, and to choose more significantly.

According to Rogers (1957) therapists must possess three qualities in order for their clients to get better. First, the therapist must show *unconditional positive regard* for the client. That is, the client must come to believe that the therapist likes and respects the client, and that this positive regard does not depend on what the client says or does. Rogers believes that unconditional positive regard from another leads to self-acceptance. Second, the therapist must show *empathic understanding*. The client must be convinced that he or she is truly understood by the therapist. In the absence of such empathic understanding, clients are likely to think, 'This therapist says he likes and respects me, but that is only because he doesn't really know me . . . if he really knew me he wouldn't like me'. Empathic understanding also helps clients get in touch with thoughts and feelings which they denied in the past. Third, the therapist must show *genuineness* – the client must perceive the therapist as honest and straightforward. If the therapist says one thing but somehow communicates contrary feelings, the client will pick this up and come to believe the therapist cannot be trusted.

In short, a therapist must show a client unconditional regard, empathy, and genuineness or the client will not get better. Rogers thinks these three attributes are sufficient to encourage psychological growth in another person. However, he may have been overoptimistic in his belief in these three conditions.

But note how the process does appear to depend upon the conditions. The unconditional positive regard, in particular, on the part of the therapist enables the client to express his feelings openly so that natural processes can work. The therapist's empathy and congruence enable him to perceive accurately the thoughts and feelings of the client, and hence make it possible for him to aid in the process of articulation. The emphasis is on the patient 'doing it by himself' (client-centred, non-directive). Rogers assumes that humans have an 'inherent tendency . . . to develop all . . . capacities in ways which serve to maintain or enhance' the person (1959, p. 196). This actualizing tendency, in reference to the self (self-actualization), means essentially a striving towards congruence between self and experience. The person, indeed, would obtain congruence on his own were it not for the denials and distortions of experience caused by the threat to self-image, and the anxiety produced by incongruence. This is the job of the therapist, in Rogers' view: 'to make these distortions unnecessary through continuing unconditional regard'.

The outcome of the therapeutic process is indicated by the process itself. The client becomes more congruent, less defensive and less anxious. His perception of himself and his experience becomes more accurate. He is more confident, indeed, more capable, and he experiences more positive self-regard. His ideal self, that 'self' on which he places the highest value, becomes more realistic; his 'real' self and his ideal self become more congruent. In short, the client would be described by an outside observer as more mature and better adjusted.

EVALUATION

Carl Rogers has provided a workable, clearly defined psychotherapeutic approach based on humanist–existential principles. The therapy is popular, and its underlying approach has had wide influence in counselling, social work and education. Client-centred therapy tends to be briefer than psychoanalysis, therefore less expensive, and the training of client-centred therapists requires considerably less time and expense. Once a week for a year or less – is commonly the case. This abbreviation has another advantage. It tends to thwart the development of complicating feelings such as the transference, and thereby fosters the positive climate Rogers so esteems.

The Rogerians take a more optimistic view of man than other therapists. The actualizing tendency is fundamentally a constructive, positive force leading to healthy and socially adaptive ways of behaving. Accurate or not, this is certainly a more positive approach and view of man. Rogerian therapy is designed for a wide spectrum of emotional states. People from the relatively normal end have worked with it, as have hospitalized neurotics. This range probably derives from its pre-occupation with problems of self-regard. Since these are universal, almost anyone can find some point of personal reference in Rogers' approach. The therapy would seem to be especially well suited for counselling people in times of stress, when the environmental situation is not in itself over-whelming but where it brings out self-defeating feelings of inferiority or insecurity – e.g. students adjusting to school. Others who could be helped by this approach are the relatively non-neurotic people of the middle classes who are experiencing loneliness and isolation as a result of alien-ation. Whether this is the best they can do to combat such feelings is another matter; but there is no doubt that Rogerian treatment applies to them.

But it does appear that this method – like psychoanalysis – can function successfully only with individuals who are fairly verbal, and are motivated to discuss their problems. With persons who do not voluntarily seek help, with normal children, and with psychotics who are too withdrawn to be able to discuss their feelings, more directive methods are usually necessary. The techniques of client-centred therapy would seem appropriate, in counselling neurotic patients, in play therapy with children (Axline) and in group therapy, with adolescents and adults in temporary crises.

It is somewhat surprising to note the many possibilities for research on Rogers' theory, given the mystical tone of its constructs. It is a tribute, of course, to Rogers' continual efforts to create workable scientific constructs without destroying the distinctive humanity of his theory.

On the level of the individual, the theory tends to phrase problems in a language system that the client can understand because he uses it in his everyday life. For example, some theories point to an event in the client's past and say in effect, 'That is why you are what you are now'. It is a psychological commonplace to say some such thing as, 'You grew up in a slum, so therefore you feel inferior today'. The client often can accept and understand such a deterministic explanation, but it gives him no basis for future action: 'O.K. so what do I do now?'

Rogers' theory, on the other hand, places full reponsibility upon the individual. It says, 'You have within you the power to change your life. It's up to you to do so. Not me, the therapist, and not the environment. You.' In Rogers' words:

> We have frequently observed that when the individual has been authoritatively told that he is governed by certain factors or conditions beyond his control, it makes therapy more difficult, and it is only when the individual discovers for himself that he can organize his perceptions that change is possible. In veterans who have been given their own psychiatric diagnosis, the effect is often that of making the individual feel that he is under an unalterable doom, that he is unable to control the organization of his life. When, however, the self sees itself as capable of reorganizing its own perceptual field, a marked change in basic confidence occurs . . . A veteran at the conclusion of counseling puts it more briefly and more positively: 'My attitude toward myself is changed now to where I feel I can do something with my self and my life.' He has come to view himself as the instrument by which some reorganization can take place (1947, pp. 361–62).

The impression of a totally client-centred method would however be misleading. The reflected verbalizations, head nods, smiles, etc. from the therapist are as striking an example of positive reinforcement à la Skinner as can be found in behaviour modification procedures. There is no doubt that even client-centred therapists encourage certain lines of verbalization and attitude expression, while extinguishing others. Even non-directive counselling must be a reinforcement process since social influence is being brought to bear however subtly on the client, simply by virtue of the therapist being there. The therapist must have an effect on the client, especially as the latter knows that the former has the title role of counsellor. But even more potent is the act of taking up one topic and allowing another to fade away, in influencing reinforcing and directing the learning of the client about himself and about what is deemed important in his life style.

Many writers criticize the vagueness of Rogers' sole drive, self-actualization, and argue that a more accurate way of expressing this promotion of client 'growth' is increasing the capacity of the client to learn. This fits in with the view above that even client-centred therapists shape, reinforce and extinguish client behaviour in all sorts of subtle ways.

Dollard and Miller (1950) argue:

> We agree with Rogers that faith in the patient is a most important requirement in a therapist. But we would describe it as a capacity to learn rather than one in a capacity to grow because 'growth' suggests physiological models which we do not believe are as appropriate or specific as the principles and conditions of learning. When we affirm the patient's capacity to learn we mean always 'provided the right conditions are set up'. Learning is not inevitable.

Shoben (1949) too writes:

> Rogers describes the therapeutic process as a freeing of the 'growth capacities' of the individual, which permits him to acquire 'more mature' ways of reacting. If 'growth' in this context means (as it must) something more than physiological maturation . . . it must refer to the client's acquisition of new modes of response. Such new modes of response are 'more mature' because for a given patient they are less fraught with anxiety or conflict. Thus Rogers is actually talking about psychotherapy as a learning process.

Truax and Corkhuff (1967) deliberately conceptualized psychotherapy as a learning experience. Hence what Rogers vaguely and mystically calls growth, can be operationalized precisely as new learning. So even the interactions of a client-centred therapist and his client may be conceptualized from a learning theory standing though the shaping, reinforcement and extinction is less overt, and deliberately planned. But it all facilitates certain learning processes viz.

(1) reinforcing positive aspects of the patient's self-concept, modifying the existing self-concept and thus leading to changes in the patient's own self-reinforcement system

(2) reinforcing self-explanatory behaviour, thus eliciting self-concepts and anxiety-laden material which can potentially be modified

(3) extinguishing anxiety or fear responses associated with specific cues, both those elicited by the relationship with the therapist and those elicited by patient self-exploration

(4) reinforcing human relating, encountering or interacting, and to extinguish fear or avoidance learning associated with human relating.

What is being created in the therapy situation is a context in which the client is positively encouraged to talk and think about himself in favourable ways, in which self denigration and emotional expression are allowed to issue forth without criticism or condemnation and so be extinguished, and in which the very experience of being able to talk to someone in a close relationship provides conditions for generalizing this activity with its overtones of personal acceptance, satisfaction and confidence building to other social situations. All this facilitates the client behaving more constructively in his day to day life.

The most important limitation of all Rogers' work is the tendency to over-emphasize the importance of therapist conditions, and the consequent lack of importance attached to treatment technique variables, the nature of the patient's psychological difficulties, and, of course, the combination and interaction of these two determinants.

The three necessary and sufficient conditions for therapeutic change, viz. genuineness, empathy and unconditional positive regard, were promoted by Rogers (1957) without equivocation. It was a bold step to argue that constructive personality change in all types of psychotherapy can only be effected when the therapist is genuine, empathic and warm. He went so far as to claim that if one or more of these conditions is not present then constructive personality change will not occur. He further argued that the techniques of the various therapies are relatively unimportant, except to the extent that they can serve as channels for fulfilling at least one of the necessary conditions. However, it would appear that these three conditions are not sufficient. Two other conditions, self-exploration and persuasive potency, have been added (Truax, 1968). Other evidence from Truax and Carkhuff (1967) reveal therapeutic change even when one of the original three conditions was negligible.

Lambert et al. (1978) pointed out that in 14 important studies reported since 1971, less than 33 per cent of the predicted relationships have been confirmed. To take one example only, they claim that in 109 tests of the relationship between empathy and outcome, only 24 were significantly positive. One of the most disappointing results was reported by Mitchell, et al. (1977) In their ambitious study of the work of 75 therapists with 120 clients, only 52 of the 1600 hypotheses tested produced a significant result! On the influence of accurate empathy, only 2 out of 562 analyses were positive. In the controlled trial carried out by Sloane *et al.* (1975) the supposedly effective therapist variables were found to be unrelated to therapy outcome, and it is amusing to observe that the behaviour therapists were found to offer more favourable therapist conditions on three out of the four scales than did the psychotherapists (Sloane *et al.*, 1975, p. 167).

A large number of studies of client-centred therapy have produced disappointing results. In 1967 Rogers and his colleagues produced a massive report on a treatment trial carried out on 16 schizophrenic patients. The therapeutic results were disappointing. The treated patients did not do better than the untreated controls. The patients who experienced high levels of the three crucial therapist conditions did not necessarily do better than those patients who experienced low levels of these conditions. Difficulties occurred in assessment. It was found, for example, that the scales for measuring one of the three conditions had a reliability which was so low that it precluded any useful result. It was also found that the therapists' assessments of their own behaviour differed significantly from that perceived by the patient or by an independent assessor. Rogers perhaps made a choice of patient for the study as schizophrenics appear less susceptible anyway to this sort of treatment than neurotics. Four recent reviews of Rogerian psychotherapy (Mitchell *et al.*, 1977; Gomez-Schwartz *et al.*, 1978; Bergin, 1975, and Lambert *et al.*, 1978) all suggest that the claims for the potency of the facilitative conditions in determining therapy outcome are not clearly supported by the evidence.

The Rogerian work has served the important function of preparing the ground for an improved understanding of the way in which a therapist can facilitate the treatment process, but continued neglect of the treatment technique and the psychological problem presented is likely to retard rather than facilitate our understanding of the contribution made by the conditions which the therapist offers.

Another major problem with Rogers' phenomenological approach comes with the use of defensive processes to cope with a state of incongruity between the organism's experience and the existing self-concept. Rogers regards behaviour as an attempt to maintain consistency of the self-concept. Hence in response to a state of incongruence, i.e. a threat presented by recognition of experience that are in conflict with the self-concept, the individual will employ one of two defensive processes. Distortion is used to alter the meaning of the experience and denial removes the existence of the experience. Rogers emphasizes the former, since if denial leaves an experience completely unsymbolized how can a phenomenological approach ever deal with such a process, since phenomenology does not accept the role of the unconscious in determining behaviour? Behaviour is simply a function of experience which leaves no place for non-conscious (unsymbolized) effects. How can a person, therefore, defend, deny or distort an experience which phenomenologically is never sensed. This is obviously a theoretical point which is not crucial to practitioners who are rightly concerned only with the effectiveness of the approach.

Other critics of this approach (e.g. Bandura, 1969) object that regardless of the client's complaints, the treatment is always the same (the same criticism has been levelled at psychoanalysis). Some contend that providing the client with 'unconditional positive regard' may actually be harmful, as clients may leave therapy with the unrealistic expectation that anything they do will meet with society's approval. It fails to take account of the real environment and the negative aspects of human needs and drives. Its supreme optimism blinds it to any recognition of the full range of human behaviour. It is solely a simple inspirational attack on a client's negative self-images using the therapist's positive regard. Behaviourists are critical of client-centred therapy as it lacks clearly defined goals specifically delineated that will lead to particular behaviour changes in the client. But this approach has been part of a significant effort to come to terms with human experience, by seeking to take behaviour as it is.

Further Reading

Burns, R. B. (1979). *The Self Concept.* (London: Longmans)

Burns, R. B. (1982). *Self Concept Development and Education.* (London: Holt, Rinehart and Winston)

Rogers, C. R. (1942). *Counseling and Psychotherapy.* (Boston: Houghton Mifflin)

Rogers, C. R. (1951). *Client-Centered Therapy.* (Boston: Houghton Mifflin)

Rogers, C. R. (1956). Client-centered therapy: A current view. In Fromm-Reichmann, F. and Moreno, J. L. (eds.) *Progress in Psychotherapy.* (New York: Grune & Stratton)

Rogers, C. R. (1959). A theory of therapy, personality and interpersonal relationships, as developed in the client-centered framework. In Koch, S. (ed.) *Psychology: A study of science.* (New York: McGraw-Hill)

Rogers, C. R. (1961). *On Becoming a Person.* (London: Constable)

Rogers, C. R. (1980). *A Way of Being.* (Boston: Houghton Mifflin)

Chapter 15

ENCOUNTER GROUPS

THEORY

Encounter groups cannot really be encapsulated under one heading, because they grow wild, proliferating on their eclectic approach to theory, order and systemization. Hence the resistance to scientific investigation that affects so much of therapy is vigorously championed again here by encounter group proponents. Because of their strong emphasis on personal growth, Lewin's T Group evolved into encounter groups as a form of group psychotherapy.

Encounter groups, also known as sensitivity groups, consist of 8–20 individuals who may meet for only one intensive weekend session or for sessions over a period of several months, in an attempt to better understand how they behave in their interpersonal interactions. Members are urged to express attitudes and feelings not usually displayed in public. The group leader (or facilitator, as he or she is sometimes called, because the job is not really to lead) encourages the participants to explore their own feelings and motives as well as those of other group members. The objective is to stimulate an exchange that is not inhibited by defensiveness, and that achieves a maximum of openness, honesty and personal authenticity to learn more honest ways of communicating with each other. Often the focus is on some aspect of non-verbal experience – perhaps on developing better sensory awareness of bodily reactions, perhaps on learning how facial expressions communicate deep-seated emotions. As a means of helping group members strip away their defences, or urging them to 'let it all hang out', a few encounter groups meet in the nude! The common features then of encounter groups are communication and exchange of feeling by physical contact, activity and non-verbal interaction generally; emphasis on intensity of present experience rather than intellectual understanding or concern with past or

170

future; and a lack of artificial barriers so that leaders are expected to set an example of openness and emotional display rather than to remain detached. Interest in certain Eastern religious ideas, particularly Zen Buddhism, has also been an important feature contributing to the abolition of artificial barriers and hierarchies.

The encounter group is not for the client seeking help with an emotional disturbance, but is the refuge of normal persons who desire more meaning, spontaneity and joy in their lives. Such clients join up, hopefully, to add something positive to their humdrum daily lives, rather than to eliminate something negative.

The Encounter group is seen by its proponents as a way of providing a middle class of frustrated, bored, dissatisfied, unhappy persons with experiences that add to the quality of their lives. Ordinary life involves tension as the constraints of living in society require the suppression of some feelings and desires.

TECHNIQUES

The general encounter group goal is not to work on specific problem areas of the members but rather to sensitize each member to the feelings of others. Members are placed in a face-to-face encounter under instructions to say what they feel and 'pull no punches'. Theoretically this procedure enables members to experience and express their feelings more forcefully.

The encounter group process varies tremendously from one group to the next. All encounter groups focus on here-and-now feelings, negative and positive feedback to each member of the group, and the removal of facades that interfere with honest, open communication. Most group leaders use a variety of techniques that are designed to make the participants communicate honestly. Some of these techniques are:

(1) Self-description. All group members write down the three adjectives most descriptive of themselves. The slips of paper are mixed, and the group discusses the kind of person that is being described.

(2) Eyeball-to-eyeball. This technique involves two participants staring into each other's eyes for a minute or two, communicating as much as possible, and discussing the feelings afterward.

(3) The blind walk. All group participants pair off, and with one person leading and the other blind-folded, the 'blind' person walks around the room or outdoors and sensitizes himself to the environment. One variant of this exercise is for the 'blind' persons to try to communicate by touch alone.

(4) Trusting exercises. Participants take turns being lifted and passed around a circle formed by the group members.

(5) Hot seat. One group member sits in a special chair, and others give the individual honest feedback about how he or she affects them.

(6) Positive and negative bombardment. In this method, similar to the hot seat technique, the group member is given feedback that focuses on only positive or only negative feedback.

Some groups may not use any formal techniques. Instead, the group is allowed to develop its own strategies for encouraging honest and open interactions.

Marathon groups

A marathon group is an encounter group in which members meet for many consecutive hours. Weekend marathons may start on Friday night and continue until Sunday night. Short breaks for eating and sleeping may be taken, but usually only in the location of the marathon. Because the weekend defines the entire encounter for the group, there is no time for group members to be supportive and tactful toward one another. There is tremendous group pressure for self-disclosure and genuine open interactions with others. The fatigue of constant group interaction tends to break down defences, making it more difficult to play those roles that often get in the way of honest communication and self-knowledge.

Sensitivity training groups

Sensitivity training, one of the popular types of encounter groups, originated as a series of group exercises designed to help business persons improve managerial skills, human relations and productivity. People were taught in an actual group experience how interpersonal relationships work, how to understand organizational behaviour, how to facilitate group functioning, and how to confront individuals with feedback about how others see them and to pressure them to exchange socially unacceptable interactions for appropriate behaviours.

The sequence of events in an encounter group is characteristic of Rogers' non-directive approach. Rogers, who has studied various types of encounter groups, describes a fairly consistent pattern of change as the sessions progress (Rogers, 1970). Initially there tends to be confusion, with a lot of defensive cocktail party talk and some frustration when the facilitator makes it clear that he or she will not take the responsibility for directing the group. There is also resistance to expressing feelings; if one member describes some personal feeling, other members may try to stop the person, questioning whether it is appropriate to express such feelings in the group. At the next stage, the participants gradually begin to talk about feelings and problems they have encountered outside the group. They then begin to discuss relationships within the group; often the first feeling expressed is a negative attitude toward oneself or toward another group member. When the individual finds that these feelings are accepted, a climate of trust begins to develop. By the final sessions, the group members have become impatient with defensiveness; they attempt to undercut facades, insisting that individuals be themselves. The tact and polite cover-up that are acceptable outside the group are not tolerated within it.

The unwelcomed honesty of the feedback enables individuals to take fuller stock of themselves and their behaviour. The counterbalancing sympathy and acceptance, sometimes with help extended outside the group situation, allows the increasing expression of closeness, affection and gratitude. The real emotional and intellectual contact in the 'here and now' is what is meant by basic encounter.

EVALUATION

The encounter group allows the removal of the ordinary constraints against what we feel to be forbidden. The group not only gives permission, it forces expression, by demanding blunt frankness or openness. To be open means just that: to do one's thing, to express one's impulse, whether it was to disrobe, curse or criticize. And this is backed up by the whole range of reinforcing tactics which give the movement its immense variety: caressing, arm-wrestling, screaming, nudity, etc. If something promotes expression of what has been held back, it will appear in some encounter group somewhere. They all function by imposing a kind of liberating imperative. In this state, feelings of intimacy may be heightened, with deep bonds of affection for co-members and veneration for the charismatic leader. The person may even learn something new about the social face he presents to the world. The reduction of defensiveness allows communication to open up, with new ideas and innovations being welcomed rather than feared. Individuals learn to discard their masks and discover their hidden selves.

Encounter experiences may allow some participants to learn more about themselves and be more honest with others. However, there are some notable disadvantages. Firstly, the frankness that pervades the ethos – no matter how laudable – does not allow for the elucidation and working through of deep-seated conflicts. Some participants may simply be made more aware of their shortcomings. Frankness does not even imply that a person is being 'open'. All that emerges is what is in the conscious mind, what is left after suppression and repression have creamed off the most succulent thoughts. It is possible to be frank and unrevealed at the same time. Secondly, such frankness, spontaneity and openness cannot be transferred in full bloom from the encounter group context to everyday life where our childhood conditioning holds impulses in check (*cf* Freudian superego), so that reasonable accommodation in social life can be met. Encounter groups reverse the balance as the former suppressed impulses are now designated 'good'. The group acceptance of such impulses allows the individual to bypass his conscience – pleasure is in, guilt is out. This is the disarming and beguiling appeal of encounter groups. But such openness and spontaneity has to be restricted to the encounter group context, for such bacchanalian indulges cannot be carried over into everyday life in the same way as behaviour learnt in rival therapies is meant to be, without destroying both self and society. Daily life is a compromise and conscience is only temporarily dimmed in 'encounter' activity. When it emerges from the shadows it is as impervious as ever, leading some clients into even greater self-punitive misery, in the anticlimax of real life.

Thirdly, the intensity of self-awareness provided so lavishly from others can lead to casualties. The demands of the encounter ethos can hurt a vulnerable person who becomes a target for others in the group. Yalom and Lieberman (1972) found that 12 per cent of Stanford University undergraduates who completed encounter groups could be considered ' "casualties" – defined as an enduring, significant, negative outcome . . . caused by their participation in the group'. This was a careful study, using selected, supposedly competent leaders representing most major therapeutic ideologies. Significantly – in the light of the propensity of therapeutic ideologues to claim wondrous results for their techniques – the authors found that 'the leader's ratings were a highly inaccurate mode of identifying casualties'.

Given the high rate of casualties and their seriousness (three students became psychotic in Yalom and Lieberman's study) one should think *thrice* before endorsing encounter groups. This is not to say that disasters do not befall other therapies. They do, but less frequently. An uncharitable view is that the encounter group imposes a tyranny of 'awareness' narrowly turned to the demands of the fellow members for a brief period. No-one should enter into encounter group activities 'just to see what goes on' or 'to have a bit of fun'. What goes on may be you, and the fun can soon turn into threatening qualms of self intimidation, self mistrust and self derogation. Only the emotionally stable should indulge themselves in the temporary unveiling of their normally hidden sides. Encounter groups are no answer to the person with a neurotic disturbance; his conflict is more than likely to worsen in response to the encounter environment. No-one needs a licence to run an encounter group so some totally unqualified and unscrupulous people have run groups, and some group members have been pushed beyond breaking point.

Unfortunately, the anti-establishment emphasis of the encounter movement has resulted in a surge of 'do-it-yourself' groups, with increasingly irresponsible experimentation. This uncontrolled development, encouraged by a naive, messianic quality in the writings of some of its leading exponents, may regretfully discredit what in the right hands is a valuable process. As Patterson (1977) argues, these innovations may be anti-therapeutic; he writes,

> Anything goes now in psychotherapy . . . Every few months we have a new technique or approach being advocated in books and journal articles. But what is discouraging – and disturbing – is the lack of, or the inadequacy of, theory and concepts supporting the new methods or techniques; the ignoring, or ignorance of, the research supporting what have come to be known as the core conditions; the evangelistic fervour with which many of the approaches are advocated; the lack of concern for any evidence of their effectiveness except possibly testimonials; the failure to recognize that what is called counselling or psychotherapy can be for better or worse – that people can be hurt as well as helped; and finally the eagerness with which the approaches are commercialized. Many of the originators of new approaches are not satisfied with publishing books and articles, and then waiting for their ideas to be subjected to critical scrutiny, evaluation and research before eventually being accepted or rejected, or modified and revised and finally incorporated in the teaching and training programmes of universities. Instead, many of these methods are being promoted by advertising and workshops and short-term training courses, or are the basis for institutes or organisations which issue diplomas and certificates, all resembling the development of a cult.

Further reading

Lieberman, L., Yalom, I. and Miles, B. (1973). *Encounter Groups. First Facts*. (New York: Basic Books)

Rogers, C. R. (1973). *Encounter Groups*. (Harmondsworth: Penguin)

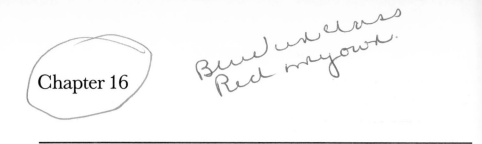

Chapter 16

GESTALT THERAPY

INTRODUCTION

Like most systems of psychotherapy, Gestalt therapy is the creation of a single individual, in this case a German-born psychologist and psychiatrist Fritz Perls (1893–1970). Perls trained as a psychoanalyst, but soon he became dissatisfied. His attempts to change psychoanalysis were not well received by his fellow psychiatrists, so he rejected psychoanalysis and began to develop his own approach. The label Gestalt therapy first appeared in 1951 (Perls, Hefferline and Goodman, 1951) although the first major workshop in Gestalt did not occur until 1963, the year Perls settled in Big Sur (Esalen), in northern California.

The term Gestalt is not entirely translatable but is perhaps best described as a meaningful organized whole or as a configuration. The 'figure' and the 'ground' are the two primary concepts delineated in the theory. Whatever is the present focus of one's attention is the figure, while all other elements of the environment at that moment make up the ground. This conception of an individual's perception of his or her world becomes important in Gestalt therapy for understanding a client's problems, as well as his or her basic auditory or visual perception. The Gestalten (plural of Gestalt) of an individual can be strong or firm, meaning that he is capable of differentiating clearly figure and ground, can use selective perception to focus on specific elements, can use motor activity directed at satisfaction of a specific need, and then can shift to a new Gestalt and new activity. Gestalt therapy emphasizes the integrating qualities of the individual within his own world. Any situation, including a person, must be understood as a whole, and the whole is always more than the sum of its parts. It is the concentration on integration and the whole that was especially helpful as an analogy to the Gestalt therapists.

Essentially, Gestalt therapists have used some of the basic concepts of Gestalt psychology and applied them to an individual's perceptions of emotions and bodily sensations.

THE THEORY

Gestalt therapists give a view of human personality that strikingly resembles the views of Carl Rogers. Thus people possess a self-actualizing tendency, which tends to become thwarted in the process of learning to get along in society. People learn not to be aware of much of what is going on around them and inside of them. Therefore, the goal of therapy is to help them learn to become more aware. Awareness is the central concept in Gestalt psychotherapy. It covers virtually everything, including our thoughts and emotions, body sensations, movements, posture, muscular tension and facial expressions, as well as an appreciation for the environment and our relationship to it. Perls wished his clients to look at the entirety of their immediate experience (the gestalt). According to Perls, people with emotional problems tend to focus their attention on only part of what they feel and on only part of what they do, especially in their communications with others. The focus of Gestalt therapy is not why the client is behaving in a certain way but rather what the person is feeling and how the person is behaving. The therapist helps the client overcome barriers to self-awareness. The goal is for the client to become aware of what he or she is doing from moment to moment, and to accept responsibility for that behaviour. Theoretically, clients will then be able to attend to all aspects of their experience. Attention and emotion, behaviour, awareness become integrated as one gestalt.

THE PRACTICE

The focus of Gestalt therapy is on the figure–ground relationship. The normal individual is well able to differentiate these two factors and the movement of them, but in a person having psychological difficulties there can be a lack of figure formation or a rigidity of a figure–ground relationship. The interplay of this figure–ground relationship is all important, and it is through understanding the problems of this relationship that the individual can come to live with less difficulty. In his or her encounter with the client, the Gestalt therapist tries to help the individual's understanding by focusing on overlooked psychological mechanisms. She shows the client how he is contradictory in his actions. Many therapists use the non-verbal behaviour of the client – movements, breathing, expressions – to aid the client in achieving better self-understanding and in completing his or her Gestalt. The therapist is attempting to remove blocks in the client's awareness of self and others, which create difficulty. She also attempts to show the client that the latter must be responsible for his own actions, no matter how trivial they may seem.

What is the value of all this awareness? A Gestalt therapist would argue that when people are not aware of what they want at any given moment, or how they are feeling, or what they are doing, the control they exercise over their feelings and behaviour is limited. At such times, they tend to do things out of habit rather than choice, and such habits are often self-defeating. For instance, a person may habitually stand 5 or 6 inches from other people when he talks to them. He is clearly not aware that he 'crowds' people, and this is unfortunate because some people avoid him for this reason. A Gestalt therapist would want to help him become aware of this annoying habit, so that he would then be in a position to make a free choice: change the behaviour and improve his social life, or continue to crowd others and risk their annoyance. Gestalt therapists believe that when confronted with such a choice, people choose self-actualizing or self-enhancing alternatives rather than self-defeating ones. Gestalt therapy dismisses language and intellect and focuses on emotion, sensation and movement. It is an organismic approach.

For Perls, current awareness and actualization involve the meaningful integration and harmony between a person and his environment. Neurosis was simply the unnatural clash between elements which should form a Gestalt, often between thought and feeling, an inability to harmonize these elements. Anxiety became the organism's sensing of this clash, and the struggle to attain unification of organism and environment to achieve wholeness (*cf* Freudian views of anxiety as anticipation of inner danger). So Gestalt therapists view neurosis as a behavioural warping, to ward off knowledge of the break up of the Gestalt. Guilt feelings are minimized in Gestalt therapy, and are seen by Perls as simply a projection of unverbalized resentment. The expression of such resentment is encouraged, thereby removing guilt. This narrows the gap between the objective and subjective modes, restoring wholeness and allowing the client to utilize his potential more effectively.

The cure, according to Perls, was not to put the client in touch with repressed memories as Freud claimed, but to encourage awareness of current organismic needs. The organism has the ability to put itself together, creating a person more capable of achieving his potential. The Gestalt therapist, therefore, facilitates the client to obtain greater awareness in the here and now, which leads to the fulfilment of potential inherent in the current situation with the 'natural' process of Gestalt formation taking place. Healing is promoted by encouraging active awareness.

Psychological growth is inhibited by 'unfinished business' – situations where, in the past, emotion or desire have been painfully blocked. Like Rogers, Perls believes that the important source of such blocks is childhood. But he makes no attempt to focus on the client's past. Nor does he seek to explain or ask his patients why. His focus is on the present and not on words but on feelings. 'Verbal communication is usually a lie', he writes, and exhorts his clients to 'lose his mind and find his senses'. This means expressing the actual bodily and perceptual sensations the client is experiencing at the time.

Therapist	What are you aware of now?
Client	Now I am aware of talking to you. I see the others in the room. I'm aware of John squirming. I can feel the tension in my shoulders. I am aware that I get anxious as I say this.
Therapist	How do you experience the anxiety?
Client	I hear my voice quiver. My mouth feels dry. I talk in a very halting way.

(Levitsky and Perls, 1970, p. 143)

It means not just being aware of feelings but accepting or owning that they are yours. One simple technique for this is to encourage clients to convert any expression of feeling into 'I' language:

Therapist	What do you feel?
Client	My hand is trembling.
Therapist	Can you take responsibility for that by saying 'I am trembling'?

One way of avoiding responsibility is to say 'I can't'. Perls tries to get the client to realize that this often means 'I won't'.

TREATMENT

The client–therapist relationship in Gestalt therapy is somewhat like the relationship between an apprentice and a master (Kempler, 1973). The skill or art is awareness. As the relationship develops, the therapist uses his or her awareness to facilitate the growth of awareness in the client. While there is no set formula for doing this, Perls and his followers (Levitsky and Perls, 1970) do provide guidelines for Gestalt therapy. Like client-centred therapy, Gestalt therapy emphasizes what the client is experiencing at the present moment. In contrast to psychoanalysis, the therapist is more interested in how a client feels about his mother now and less interested in what he thought and felt about her as a young child.

An important element of therapy is that the client should develop a sense of personal responsibility. Gestalt therapists believe that any action implies a choice, and with choice goes responsibility. Sometimes the therapist deliberately frustrates the client, especially when the client tries to lean on the therapist when support is not really necessary.

Joen Fagan (1970) has outlined a number of tasks that must be carried out by a Gestalt therapist. First, the therapist must come to a decision on the behaviour patterns of the client who has come to him – he must understand the problems of the client and decide how to correct them. Second, the therapist must have control in the therapy – he must be able to induce the client to follow his suggestions and procedures. However, the client also has control in the situation because he has sought therapy by choice, and because he must specify the changes which he desires in himself. Third, the therapist's techniques must be potent in order to bring about the change in the client. Fourth, the therapist must be committed to his individual clients and to work as a therapist. These tasks may be the *sine qua non* of any successful psychotherapeutic interaction, but the emphasis on these humanistic goals is noteworthy among humanistic therapists.

Perls and other Gestalt therapists felt that the therapeutic situation must be as undogmatic as possible. Explicit demands should not be made of the client, but 'experimental' situations should be set up so that he can better understand and cope with his problems. Some experimental situations for the client should be designed to help him be in contact with the environment and his awareness of it. Techniques to help the client feel the actual or to show the client opposed forces in his environment are used, so that the individual can become aware of the variety of processes which result in integrated psychological functioning. There are a number of experimental situations that are designed to aid an individual when he is not functioning properly in his environment. These are experiments involving retroflection, where the client should learn to understand misdirected activities and energies; projection, where the client understands that certain feelings really originate in him and not in others to whom he had attributed them; and introjection, where the client sees that he has been forced to accept certain aspects about himself that are really not genuine parts of himself. These experimental explorations are done gradually, one experience building on another.

The Gestalt approach is usually conducted in groups, and undertaken in an intensively concentrated workshop setting rather than regular meetings over a period of time. This leads to more dramatic results, particularly as participants are encouraged to enact their conflicts dramatically in the therapeutic theatre rather than simply verbalize them. Expression is encouraged rather than simple explanation.

The dramatization employs various rules (Levitsky and Perls, 1972). The major principles are those of (1) 'Now', where the 'why' of remote causation is rejected in favour of concentrating awareness on current feelings completely, (2) 'I and Thou' where clients are urged to talk at rather than to others, (3) 'No Gossiping' so that the others must be addressed directly and not talked about as though *in absentia* and (4) 'No It Language', so that when people talk about parts of their body they have to translate 'it' into 'I' language, for example, 'my tummy is tense' becomes 'I am tense'. Similarly, passive expressions like 'It was annoying' becomes 'I am annoyed at myself'.

The dramatical enactments occur during various exercises.

Empty chair exercise, here the client moves back and forth physically between two chairs. In one of the two chairs, the client assumes his or her own role. In the other chair, the client assumes the role of another person, perhaps a parent or a spouse. Clients also can use the two chairs to represent two conflicting aspects of themselves. For example, a client reported that whenever she thought about her deceased father she became anxious and confused. She was asked to imagine her father in the empty chair and to tell him what she resented in him. In a minute or two she was telling her imagined father, in a very emotional tone of voice, that she could never forgive him for dying without ever telling her he loved her and was proud of her. She was then asked to sit in the other chair and reply as her father would. The 'father' was also emotional, saying in a sad, tearful way that he had indeed loved his daughter, but that he had never been able to express his feelings, because men were not supposed to be emotional. At the end of the exercise, the client said that she felt more 'together' about her father.

Making the rounds involves the client in replacing a general remark about the group by a process of addressing the remark individually to each in turn, or translating it into more emotional body language (for example, caressing, or giving vent to hostility).

Unfinished business refers to bringing into the treatment situation, and facing directly there, unresolved feelings from the client's earlier life, for example about parents or siblings.

Amplification is another exercise, where the therapist asks the client to exaggerate some behaviour or feeling in order to become more aware of it. For instance, a certain client always talked about his wife in glowing terms, but the therapist noticed that at the same time, the client tended to draw his fingers toward his palm ever so slightly. When asked to exaggerate what he was experiencing, the client made a fist and struck the table, saying, 'Why does she have to put me down all the time?'

Gestalt therapists also have the clients play different roles from their dreams to come to a better understanding of these parts of themselves, and to integrate the fragmented aspects both intellectually and emotionally. If, for example, a person dreams of a lonely tramp, the therapist would ask him or her to play that tramp experiencing the feelings of loneliness and rejection, and by doing this capture some of his or her feelings about being deserted by others, unacceptable, and alone. The therapist's job is mainly to catalyse awareness. Though he is generally quite active, he keeps himself offstage, in the prompter's box. All is referred to the client. For example, if the client feels criticized by the therapist, he is urged to play the therapist and utter aloud the criticism he has been imagining. Similarly figures from the past, and images from dreams and fantasies, are played out by the client. No comment about, no reference to, is tolerated; everything must be dealt with here, now, and with as much full being as the patient can muster. Perls called his approach to dreams the 'identification' technique, but the term applies as well to the therapy as a whole. To bring split-off projections back to the self – 'You are you and I am I', goes Perls' 'Gestalt Prayer' – and to let the self identify with and accept all its urgings and sensations – this is the core of the Gestalt method. Of course, the goal of Gestalt therapy is not simply to help the client become aware of some specific thing, but rather to teach the client how to become aware, so that the client may do this independently. When this goal has been achieved, therapy is complete.

Notice in the following excerpt of a Gestalt group therapy session how the therapist points out all aspects of the client's behaviour – the tone of her own voice and the shaking of her leg. The client had been describing a dream in which her dead mother appeared, and the therapist, noticing that she was beginning to sound whiny and complaining, asked her if she had any 'unfinished business' with her mother. The client replied:

MRS R: Well . . . if only she had loved me, things would be different. But she didn't and . . . and I've never had any real mother love. (crying)

T:	Put your mother in that chair and say that to her.
MRS R:	If only she had cared for me, I'd be much better today.
T:	I want you to say this to her, not to me. Can you imagine her sitting there in front of you?
MRS R:	Yes, I see her as she looked when she was still alive. Mother, if you had only loved me. Why couldn't you ever tell me you loved me? Why did you always criticize me? (almost a wail, more tears)
T:	Now switch over to the other chair and play your mother. (She moves over to the other chair and doesn't say anything.)
T:	What do you experience as your mother?
MRS R:	I-I-I don't know . . . I don't know what she would say.
T:	Of course you don't know. She's not around any more. You're playing the part of you that is your mother. Just say whatever you experience there.
MRS R:	Oh, I see. Well, I don't know what to say to her.
T:	Say that to her.
MRS R M (MRS R AS MOTHER):	I don't know what to say to you. I never knew what to say to you. I really did love you, you know that. Look at all the things I did for you, and you never appreciated it. (voice sounds defensive and whiny)
T:	Now switch back and reply as yourself.
MRS R S (MRS R AS SELF):	Loved me! All you ever did was criticize me. Nothing I ever did was good enough! (voice beginning to sound more whiny) When I got married to J. you disapproved, you were always coming over and telling me what I was doing wrong with the kids. Oh, you never came right out and said anything, but you were always making snide remarks or saying, 'Now, dear, wouldn't it be a good idea to put another blanket on the baby'. You made my life miserable; I was always

	worrying about you criticizing me. And now I'm having all this trouble with J. (breaks down and starts to cry.)
T:	Did you hear your voice?
MRS R S:	Yes
T:	What did you hear in it?
MRS R S:	Well, I guess I sounded kind of complaining, like I'm feeling sore – like I'm feeling mad.
T:	You sounded more like feeling self-pity. Try this on for size: say to your mother, 'Look what you've done to me. It's all your fault'.
MRS R S:	Look what you've done. Everything's your fault.
T:	Now let yourself switch back and forth as you find yourself changing roles.
MRS R M:	Come on, stop blaming me for everything. You are always complaining about something. If you had been better – if you had been a decent daughter, I wouldn't have had to criticize you so much.
MRS R S:	Oh, oh (under her breath) Damn. (She's swinging her right leg slightly.)
T:	Notice your leg.
MRS R S:	I-I'm shaking it.
T:	Exaggerate that, shake it harder.
MRS R S:	(shakes leg harder, it begins to look like a kick)
T:	Can you imagine doing that to your mother?
MRS R S:	No, but I-I-I-I'm sure feeling pissed at her.
T:	Say this to her.
MRS R S:	I feel pissed off at you! I hate you!
T:	Say that louder.
MRS R S:	I hate you! (volume higher, but still some holding back)
T:	Louder!
MRS R S:	I HATE YOU, YOU GODDAMNED BITCH. (She sticks her leg out and kicks the chair over.)
T:	Now switch back.
MRS R M:	(Voice sounds much weaker now) I-I guess I

	didn't show you much love. I really felt it, but I was unhappy and bitter. You know all I had to go through with your father and brother. You were the only one I could talk to. I'm sorry . . . I wanted you to be happy . . . I wanted so much for you.
MRS R S:	You sure did! . . . I know you did love me, Mother, I know you were unhappy. (voice much softer now, but sounding real, not whiny or mechanical) I guess I did some things that were ba – wrong, too. I was always trying to keep you off my back.
MRS R M:	Yes, you were pretty sarcastic to me too. And that hurt.
MRS R S:	I wish you had told me. I didn't think you were hurt at all.
MRS R M:	Well, that's all over now.
MRS R S:	Yeah, it is. I guess there's no use blaming you. You're not around any more.
T:	Can you forgive your mother now?
MRS R S:	Mother, I forgive you . . . I really do forgive you. (Starts crying again, but not in the whiny way of before. She sounds genuinely grieving and cries for a couple of minutes.)
T:	Now switch back.
MRS R M:	I forgive you too, dear. You have to go on now. You can't keep blaming me forever. I made my mistakes but you have your own family and you're doing okay.
T:	Do you feel ready to say goodbye now?
MRS R S:	Yes. I-I think so. (starts to sob) Goodbye, Mother, goodbye. (breaks down, cries for a few minutes)
T:	What do you experience now?
MRS R:	I feel better. I feel . . . kind of relieved, like a weight is off my back. I feel calm.
T:	Now that you've said goodbye to her, to this dead person, can you go around and say hello to the live people here, to the group?
MRS R:	Yes, I'd like that.

(She goes around the room, greets people, touches some embraces others. Many in the group are tearful. When she reaches her husband, she starts crying again, and tells him she loves him and they embrace.) (Tobin, 1971, pp. 154–5)

EVALUATION

As part of the humanist movement, Gestalt therapy can be applied to clients complaining of middle class alienation, anomie and slight to moderate neuroses. It is more emotionally demanding than Rogerian client-centred therapy and on these grounds would be less suitable for the chronic neurotic and psychotic at one extreme, and for supportive counselling at the other. Its appeal would mainly suit intellectualized neurotic clients whose personal relationships have decayed or who feel pent-up and resentful. It does require clients who are able under encouragement to open up emotionally in a group setting.

The disadvantages are firstly that the therapy can produce states of near hysteria in some clients; if the situation gets out of hand even more trouble is created for the hard pressed client. Secondly, there is an over-emphasis on emotional as against intellectual experience. Thirdly, as with all the therapies in this humanistic tradition, it is limited in application as it cannot deal with problems that are deep-seated for which a comprehensive knowledge and investigation of the individual and/or environment is necessary. Fourthly, rather strangely, though the therapy is conducted in a group setting and has an explicit social critique, group dynamics and processes sadly are not invoked in any systematic way. Other group members watch and participate vicariously on the side lines while one of their members is helped to expand his self-awareness. Finally, with Gestalt therapists, verbalizations tend to be distrusted as defensive (Perls uses the term 'bull shit'). While psychoanalysts, too, watch out for wordy defensiveness in their own practice, on the other hand they would regard total reliance on immediacy and feeling as equally defensive and misleading.

Little has been done to validate Gestalt therapy with well-controlled research. We simply do not know whether Gestalt therapy is effective or not. Gestalt therapists, like certain psychoanalysts, argue (like Freud) that we do not need controlled research, because the direct personal experience of so many clients provides such convincing evidence that the treatment works! Many Gestalt therapists also argue that their treatment is so individualized it simply cannot be put to the same experimental tests used with more standardized techniques. These pro-Gestalt arguments will hardly sway those psychologists who insist on rigorous experimental validation. Clearly, this debate is not likely to see a speedy resolution.

Gestalt therapy has the flavour of an existential approach. However, it lacks the despair that characterizes the European analysis of 'being-in-the-world' and takes on a positive American ethos that growth and enhancement are possibilities within us all given the appropriate conditions in which the blocks of resentment, hurt and needs can be openly and publicly expressed. In Perls' words:

> ... anyone who has a little bit of good will benefit from the gestalt approach because the simplicity of the gestalt approach is that we pay attention to the obvious, to the utmost surface. We don't delve into a region which we don't know anything about, into the so-called 'unconscious'. I don't believe in repressions (*sic*). The whole theory of repression is a fallacy. We can't repress a need. We have only repressed certain expressions of these needs. We have blocked one side, and then the self-expression comes out somewhere else, in our movements, in our posture, and most of all in our voice. A good therapist doesn't listen to the content of the bullshit the patient produces, but to the sound, to the music, to the hesitations. Verbal communication is usually a lie. The real communication is beyond words. (1969, p. 57)

Gestalt therapy has a transcendental quality in its beliefs in the unity of all experience and the inherent goodness of man, providing almost an American strain of some Eastern religion. This is evident in Perls' Gestalt Prayer, which emphasizes, some would argue, in a rather cold and dispassionate tone that individuals should take responsibility for themselves rather than for each other.

> I do my thing and you do your thing.
> I am not in this world to live up to your expectations
> And you are not in this world to live up to mine.
> You are you and I am I,
> And if by chance we find each other, it's beautiful.
> If not, it can't be helped.
>
> (Perls, 1969, p. 4)

Many satirical versions of this 'prayer' have been written to bring out the implicit lack of warmth in personal relationship that Perls appears to be advocating. One version runs as follows:

> I do my laundry and you do yours.
> I am not in this world to listen to your ceaseless yammering,

And you are not in this world for any discernible reason at all.
You are you, and I am I, and I got the better deal.
And if by chance we find each other, it will be unspeakably tedious.
F . . . off.

(Carroll, in Greening, 1977)

Further reading

Fagan, J. and Shepherd, I. (eds.) (1970). *Gestalt Therapy Now: Theory, Techniques, Applications.* (New York: Science and Behaviour Books)

Perls, F. S. (1969). *Gestalt Therapy Verbatim.* (Lafayette, California: Real People Press)

Perls, F., Hefferline, R. F. and Goodman, P. (1951). *Gestalt Therapy.* (New York: Julian Press)

Perls, F. (1974). *Gestalt Therapy Integrated.* (New York: Vintage Books)

Chapter 17

TRANSACTIONAL ANALYSIS

INTRODUCTION

Of all the recent outpourings of therapy in the last two decades, transactional analysis or TA is the all American smash hit with Eric Berne's *Games People Play* (1964) and Thomas Harris' *I'm OK - You're OK* (1967) becoming best sellers.

TA was the brainchild of Eric Berne, who was originally a Freudian psychoanalyst. He branched out into group therapy and developed a psychological shorthand for describing transactions (structured reciprocal interactions) between people in groups. Adler and Sullivan rather than Freud permeate the tone and ethos of TA. Transactional analysis can be described as a system with which we can analyse all personal and interpersonal communication and behaviour. The simple model that Berne evolved can be used to describe all the information that is exchanged in everyday living.

THE THEORY

TA has its own terminology, with 'Strokes' as environmental responses often from others. OK and not-OK postures are feelings of security, and self-esteem or inferiority and self doubt. Analysis of the ego and consciousness (the Parent, Adult, and Child - 'P-A-C' - ego states) are involved rather than infantile sexuality and the repressed unconscious. Transactional Analysis focuses on the ego and on consciousness because these concepts explain and predict behaviour more effectively than do psychoanalytic concepts.

The central thesis of TA, as Harris teaches it, stems from Alfred Adler's concept of a universal 'inferiority feeling'. Most people, Harris says, never stop thinking of themselves as helpless children overwhelmed by the power of adults. For that reason they go through life believing that they are inferior, or 'not OK', while they view everyone else as superior, or 'OK'. The aim of TA therapy is to instill the conviction that 'I'm OK – you're OK', meaning that no one is really a threat to anyone else.

> Every human being is born a prince or princess; early experiences convince some that they are frogs and the rest of the pathological development follows from this. (Berne, 1966, p. 289)

Ego states

More specifically, transactional analysts believe that what makes a person unhappy is an unbalanced relationship between the three parts that constitute every human personality: Parent, Adult and Child. Harris rejects any suggestion that these are the equivalent of Freud's superego, ego and id. 'The Parent, Adult and Child are real things that can be validated', he insists. 'We're talking about real people, real times and real events, as recorded in the brain'. Be that as it may, the theory is that unless the mature, rational Adult dominates the personality, or, in the language of TA, is 'plugged in', the overly restrictive Parent and the primitive, self-depreciating Child will foul up most 'transactions', or relationships with others.

The Child

The focus of the therapy is the transactions that people have with one another, and how those transactions express those three basic aspects of the personality, the Child, the Parent and the Adult. According to TA, in each of us there is a Child that is made up of the residuals of our childhood way of behaving and thinking; it functions in two ways. On the one hand our Natural (or Free) Child displays emotion, is spontaneous, fantasizing and creative. It is also selfish and manipulative. The Natural Child is loud, insistent and demanding and says things like 'I want', 'give it to me now' and 'mine'. It can also be lovable, friendly, affectionate and fun-loving. Berne believed the Natural Child was the most valuable part of personality. It motivates the Adult to obtain the greatest amount of gratification for itself, by letting the Adult know what it wants and by consulting the Parent about its appropriateness. On the other hand, the Adapted Child is compliant, polite and restrained. Because the Adapted Child functions in response to external (Parent) messages, it is also seen as rebellious at times. No doubt much of the behaviour of students and trainees can be classified as being either Natural or Adapted Child.

The situation of childhood leads the child to experience feelings of frustration, rejection, or fear of abandonment, leading the child to feel 'not OK'. There are many positive sides to the Child as well. Creativity, curiosity, exploration, the ability to touch, feel and experience, and the excitement of new discoveries are all stored in the recording of the Child.

The Parent

Our Parent ego state (or frame of mind) is made up of the attitudes and behaviours each of us observed in our own parents and other influential grown-ups when we were small. Their words, tones of voice and gestures were recorded in our brain like video-recordings, to be replayed when we find ourselves in similar situations in later life.

There are two readily observable functions of this ego state. The first is to act in a controlling way; that is to say to be judgemental, arbitrary, authoritarian, to set standards and make rules. When people function in this way they operate as the Critical Parent. The Critical Parent uses words and phrases like 'you should', 'you must', 'good/bad', 'do it now', 'listen to me'. These words are usually accompanied by gestures such as finger-pointing, folded arms and hands on hips. The voice tones would tend to be hard and the facial expression stern or frowning. Besides controlling, the Parent has the function of caring for, comforting and showing concern for other people and their opinions. This is termed Nurturing Parent. It can be recognized by the warm tones of voice, non-threatening gestures, and words like 'let me', 'don't worry', and 'be careful'.

It is quite probable that teachers and trainers spend a lot of time using these behavioural modes, and are seen as either Critical or Nurturing Parents. Since the child is relatively incapable of interpreting the meaning of what is happening to him or her at this age, these recordings are made without editing (or question). The source of all rules and judgements or how-to-do-it instructions is in the Parent, and the child is unable to determine whether the rule is good (don't play with that knife!) or poor (never get dirty!). The replaying of the Parent 'tapes' later in life has a powerful influence on personality.

The Adult

The remaining ego state, the Adult, is often referred to as the computer of the personality. It deals primarily with facts and realistic data. It is not concerned with the automatic prejudices of the Parent, nor the spontaneous emotions of the Child. It asks for, stores, processes and gives out information and data. It measures alternatives and makes rational decisions. It is seen as the most desirable of the ego states.

However, this is not necessarily so. Each ego state and associated behaviours are desirable or undesirable only insofar as they are relevant to the immediate situation. A healthy, well-balanced person has access to, and uses, the different ego states as appropriate. It should also be noted that these ego states are not age-related. Everybody has three ego states, although the degree to which they use them varies from person to person.

If we consider teachers in these terms we have a very practical way of explaining their behaviour, its effect on their teaching style and relationships with their students. Theoretically, a 'good' teacher would distribute equal amounts of energy between the ego state functions, with the exception, perhaps of Adapted Child. The reality is likely to be very different, for teachers, like the rest of the population, tend to have a 'favourite' ego state which they use in preference to the others.

The relevance of this line of argument should now be apparent. The Critical Parent, for example, is necessary to us in knowing what is right and what is wrong, in setting acceptable standards, in having and passing on a moral code of practice by which to live. However, too much reliance on this ego state will interfere with, rather than promote, effective communication. In the context of a professional–client relationship, an over-authoritarian moralistic rigid style will generally invoke attitudes of over-adaptation or rebelliousness. Similarly, an excess of Nurturing Parent behaviour will have the same effect. Over-nurturing leads to a smothering of the student's growth, blocking his ability to think for himself. Again this produces over-adaptation, over-reliance and even rebelliousness.

So to summarize then, the three ego states consist of a Parent, based on the controlling behaviours, judgements and attitudes derived from our parents' treatment of us as children; an Adult, the mature, reasoning, adaptive part of personality; and the Child, the recording from early childhood of internal events: the child's reactions to what he or she sees and hears.

Transactions

Transactional analysis therapy involves using the above vocabulary to analyse the types of interactions (transactions) that people have with one another, and to help them understand the difficulties of inappropriate interactions. People can communicate with each other as Parent to Parent, Parent to Child, Parent to Adult, Child to Parent, Child to Child, Child to Adult, Adult to Parent, Adult to Child, and, finally, Adult to

Adult. This last type of transaction is the ideal and is very difficult to achieve.

Transactional therapy allows one to understand the communication interactions one is having, to listen to and appreciate one's Child and Parent, and to train the Adult to make conscious decisions that allow the Child and Parent to be expressed in behaviour in reasonable and controlled ways.

To put his Adult in charge, Harris says, the troubled person must 'learn the language of transactional analysis, and use it in examining his everyday transactions'.

Complementary transactions
So when people communicate they are speaking from, and addressing themselves to, specific ego states. When a person makes a statement he directs it to the ego state from which he expects a response. When he gets the expected response the transaction is complementary. As long as the transactions remain complementary, effective communication can continue. That is the first rule of communication. The client must also learn to diagram these transactions, using three circles to represent the personality components of each person and drawing arrows to show how two people interact. Parallel lines depict 'complementary transactions', which occur, for instance, when a husband's Adult speaks to his wife's Adult and gets a response in kind: see Figure 4. In that type of exchange, the husband might ask 'Where are my car keys?' and his wife might reply, 'In the pocket of your brown jacket' – or perhaps, 'I'm not sure, but I'll help you find them.'

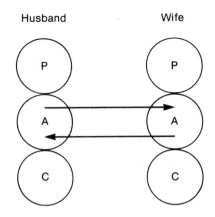

Figure 4 A complementary transaction

Crossed transactions

The second rule of communication states that when communication breaks down it is as a result of a crossed transaction; that is to say, when the response comes from an unexpected ego state (Figure 5).

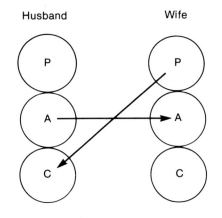

Figure 5 A crossed transaction

Crossed lines like this denote uncomplementary transactions, and bode trouble. For example, the Adult-to-Adult question about the car keys might be answered with a sharp 'Where you left them', a reproof that comes from the wife's Parent and is addressed to what she sees as the inept Child in her husband's personality. Another crossed transaction involving the husband's Child reacting sharply to what he sees as the reproving Parent in the wife is depicted in Figure 6.

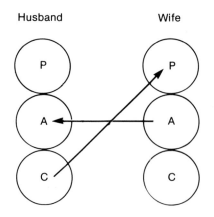

Figure 6 A crossed transaction

Ulterior transactions

The third rule of communication states that when communication is carried out at two levels, it is the psychological message that is generally acted upon. This rule refers to what are termed ulterior transactions. A transaction is ulterior when a person says one thing and means something else. The social message (that which is said) hides the unspoken psychological message (that which is implied and unsaid). Figure 7 illustrates this type of transaction, where the solid lines carry the spoken message and the dotted ones the secret message.

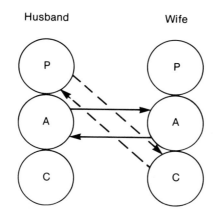

Figure 7   An ulterior transaction

Transactional analysis is a dynamic theory of personality in that it uses the concepts of psychic energy and of cathexis or distribution of energy. At a given moment the ego state which is most strongly cathected will have executive power. Berne writes of the 'flow of cathexis' which represents shifts in ego states. He considers that the most convenient way of acknowledging the differentiation of ego states is to view each state as having a boundary which separates it from other ego states. Ego states are viewed as semi-permeable under most conditions. Shifts in ego state depend on three factors: (1) the forces acting on each state, (2) the permeability of the boundaries between ego states, and (3) the cathectic capacity of each ego state. Berne observes that it is the quantitative balance between these three factors which determines the clinical condition of the patient, and thus indicates the therapeutic procedures. Berne posits that there are three principal forms of drive, hunger or motivation. First, is stimulus hunger, with the most favoured forms of stimuli being those offered by physical intimacy. The dangers of over-stimulation as well as those of under-stimulation are acknowledged. Second, there is recognition hunger, which may be viewed as a partial transformation of infantile stimulus hunger. Berne uses the term 'stroking' to denote any act implying recognition of another's presence. There are numerous rituals, such as saying 'Hello!', which imply recognition and give gratification. Biologically, even negative recognition has an advantage over no recognition at all. Third, there is structure hunger, or the everyday problem of how to structure one's waking hours. Such time structuring is concerned only with social time or the time people spend with others.

Time structuring

Berne observes that if two or more people are in a room together they have six possible kinds of social behaviour or time structuring from which to choose. These are:

(1) *Withdrawal*, here two people do not overtly communicate with one another, for example if they are on a bus or are withdrawn schizo-phrenics. In withdrawal, people remain wrapped up in their own thoughts.

(2) *Rituals*, are stylized signs of mutual recognition dictated by tradition and social custom. At the simplest level, two people saying 'Hello' would be engaging in a ritual.

(3) *Activities*, more commonly called work, are not just concerned with dealing with the material means of survival. They also have a social significance in that they offer a framework for various kinds of recognition and satisfactions. Berne considered that work trans-actions were typically Adult-to-Adult, oriented mainly towards external reality.

(4) *Pastimes*, are semi-ritualistic, topical conversations which last longer than rituals but are still mainly socially programmed. Pastimes might include 'The Weather' and 'Motor Cars'. The focus of pastimes tends to be external to the participants rather than self-referent.

(5) *Games*, in contrast to pastimes, are sequences of transactions which are based more on individual than on social programming. A psycho-logical game is a set of covert or ulterior as well as overt transactions which lead to a predictable outcome or payoff. Frequently these payoffs involve negative feelings or 'rackets' such as anger and depression. Collecting racket feelings is known as collecting 'trading stamps', which may some day be cashed in for behaviours such as a

good cry or going out and buying some new clothes. More drastically, 'trading stamps' may be cashed in for divorce or attempted suicide. Each game has a motto by which it can be recognized, for example 'Why Don't You? – Yes But' and 'If It Weren't For You'. Some of these games are discussed later.

(6) *Intimacy*, represents individual and instinctual programming in which social programming and ulterior motivations are largely, if not totally, suspended. Intimacy is the most satisfying solution to stimulus, recognition, and structure hunger, but unfortunately it is not very common for people to live as 'princes' and 'princesses'. Berne's idea of intimacy includes, but is not restricted to, sexual intimacy.

THE PROCEDURE

Berne's communication concepts can be separated into four specific areas.

Structural analysis
This deals with the structure and functions of the personality of the individual, and is the first stage of therapy. Here the client comes to observe the three individual ego states within himself, learns to recognize them in the behaviour of others, and to recognize how these ego states interact with each other.

Transactional analysis
Analysing and classifying the elements of communication between individuals; the primary purpose of transactional analysis is the gaining of social control by having the individual's Adult retain the executive control of all social situations. Other ego states would be allowed to come into interaction by the Adult, but it should remain in control. Using a technique called 'regression analysis' Berne highlights the Child in the client – he or she will re-experience phenomenologically the feelings of the Child. At this time it is not the individual's Adult talking about the Child, but instead the Child himself talking and experiencing. Berne believed that such an experience can be greatly enriched if the therapist takes over the role of the Child in him or her and interacts with the client from this position. The therapist begins the regression analysis by stating 'I am five years old and I have not yet been to school. You are whatever age you choose, but under eight. Now go ahead' (Berne, 1961, 227). The interaction then proceeds with the patient experiencing his or her own Child to

a much greater extent than if it was only spoken about. Both the therapist and patient learn about issues that affect the Child ego state as well as the person's Adult and Parent.

Even though the transactional therapist works with a wide range of psychopathologies, he or she must believe in the Adult of all patients. The therapist must also keep his patients aware of the progress they have made and where they are going.

While structural analysis is usually done in an individual setting, transactional analysis usually takes place within the context of a group, since its basic aim is control of the self in a social interaction. The patient can only learn this control within a group situation. The transactional therapist is flexible, so that he or she can also explore problems with a patient in individual sessions at any time during the therapy if the patient requests a private meeting. Following transactional analysis proper, game analysis and script analysis can be employed along with a continued use of the transactional.

Game analysis

This involves identifying and breaking up repetitive and damaging patterns of ulterior behaviour, and is useful in attaining social control. There are numerous psychological games that an individual plays, many of them destructive to that person and to the others involved in the transaction. Games appear to be like other interactions on the surface but have hidden ulterior transactions within them, and involve payoffs often not evident to those involved. The basic problem with all games is that they do not allow intimate and honest relationships to result from the interactions, and often terminate in bad feelings for at least one of the people involved. Whilst the experience of a bad feeling is uncomfortable, the recipient is getting some recognition of his existence, and negative recognition is better than none at all. In fact the need for recognition has been shown to be as necessary to human well-being as the biological need for food and drink.

Unfortunately few people are aware of either the games they initiate, or of the others into which they are drawn. This is supported by the observation that we play our games from a position of unawareness, although the feelings of discomfort at the termination of a game indicate some sense of manipulating or being manipulated. Berne gives as an example of how a game might be learned from the case of 3 year-old Mike who, when his 7 year-old brother was allowed to leave the table and lie down because of a stomach-ache said 'I have a stomach-ache too', as though he wanted the same consideration. Mike's parents, however, did not co-operate, and hence may have saved him from the game of pleading illness (social transaction) in order to gain some privilege for himself (ulterior or psychological transaction). Berne considered that games are imitative in nature.

Games are repetitive in nature, and this repetitiveness has led to the recognition of the more commonly occurring ones. These Berne listed in his book *Games People Play* (1964), each with a name which accurately describes the final outcome. Berne gave many of these games amusing titles, although in reality they are often far from funny. In pathological cases games can end in injury, mental illness or even death.

Here, briefly described are some games that are likely to be played in the learning situation.

Kick Me. Here the initiator says or does things which provoke others to criticize or punish him in some way. This negative recognition is better than no recognition at all. Kick Me players attract Critical Parent behaviour by operating from their Adapted Child ego state.

Stupid. Closely related to Kick Me. In this game the initiator needs repetitive clarification on points of misunderstanding. At the climax he may well say 'I must be stupid', unless somebody beats him to it and says it for him. People who really are stupid try to hide the fact. People playing Stupid advertise a level of stupidity they do not actually possess.

Blemish. Here the player's Critical Parent enjoys feelings of superiority by always being able to find some minute fault or blemish, no matter how well the job is performed.

Try and Make Me. This person's Rebellious Child will often provoke somebody to expend a great deal of energy in getting him to do something he has no intention of doing. Frequently recognized by the folded arms and tightly-closed mouth.

If It Weren't For You. A person can complain endlessly that if it were not for a husband, wife, child, boss or some other person, they could engage in an activity from which at present they feel restricted. Sometimes, however, these other people are being used to defend the person against the realization that, if it were not for them, he or she might be unable to perform a difficult or anxiety-evoking task. Also, if the task were performed, it would no longer be possible to cause the other person discomfort by saying, 'If It Weren't For You'. The game validates the life-position that others are Not OK.

Uproar. Many couples play Uproar in which any minor incident leads to a fight, the outcome being withdrawal on one or both member's part. The ulterior motive of the game is the avoidance of sexuality and intimacy between the couple, which is successfully accomplished by the game.

Wooden Leg. Here the person cannot possibly do what is expected because of some physical defect.

Rapo. This is where a person is first seductive and then completely unwilling, blaming the other for making advances.

Now I've got You. The initiator will watch, even set up a situation where somebody makes a mistake. He then steps in to point out the error or inconsistency, causing the other person to feel bad whilst he enjoys feelings of superiority.

Why Don't You? . . . Yes But. The initiator invites advice from others with 'I've got a problem'. This hooks their Nurturing Parent. Solutions are rejected with 'Yes But . . . ' culminating in feelings of self-righteousness at the expense of the others involved.

All of these games have different levels of intensity and most become repetitive and, therefore, even more destructive for those involved. Identifying and avoiding psychological games like these is one of the most effective applications of transactional analysis. It can lead to a more open style of communication and closer personal relationships. It also promotes feelings of improved physical and mental well-being.

Script analysis

Involves identifying the prohibitive and permissive messages around which children make lifelong decisions for living. Scripts are more than the repetition of games. They are the overall way one plays out one's life. They are usually laid down early in childhood and are greatly influenced by our culture, family and especially our parents (Berne, 1972). The problem with scripts, just as with games, is that they are limiting. Scripts restrict the aspirations and the potential of each individual. Script analysis should aid clients in seeing how, and why they are playing a role throughout their lives. For example, if an individual always snatches defeat from the jaws of victory, getting right to the point of being successful in a career and then managing to undo all of his or her hard work, this would be the script of 'Sisyphus, or There I Go Again' (Berne, 1972). The individual must learn to see this pattern in his life, and understand how it relates to parental demands placed on him many years before. He or she then has the possibility of changing the script.

Berne viewed the aim of transactional analysis as social control or autonomy, or the ability of the Adult to decide when to release the Parent or Child and when to resume the executive. If a person does not have social control, others can consciously or unconsciously activate that person's Parent or Child ego states in ways which may not be helpful.

Autonomy refers to the capacity for 'non-script' behaviour which is reversible, 'with no particular time schedule, developed later in life, and not under parental influence'. Autonomous behaviour is the opposite of script behaviour. Furthermore, autonomy consists of the active development of personal and social control so that significant behaviour becomes a matter of free choice. Berne summarizes the process of the attainment of autonomy as 'obtaining a friendly divorce from one's parents (and from other Parental influences) so that they may be agreeably visited on occasion, but are no longer dominant'. The attainment of autonomy involves the person's regaining three basic capacities of the fundamental OK position: awareness, spontaneity and intimacy.

EVALUATION

TA is short (usually small multiples of ten once-weekly sessions), to the point (a contract, faithfully obeyed, is decided upon during the first session) and educational. The leader stays close to the level of the members. There is a lot of give-and-take by everybody, good humour is encouraged and verbal exchange is the means, as the members analyse each other's 'scripts' and 'games' – which have sustained their lifelong non-OK-ness.

The attraction of TA is twofold. Firstly Berne and Harris had a talent for popular exposition, by stripping language bare of terms that referred to hidden mental phenomena, or were at a high degree of abstraction. TA aficionados like to claim that this de-mystifies psychology and gets it down to where people can use it. This is true; it is also true, however, that by means of this strategy a critical dimension is lost. The group will be bound together at the level of what is immediately evident. A de-mystified language is one in which nothing baffling can be recognized; there are no hidden meanings that can't be rapidly worked out by script analysis. Any drift towards the repressed unconscious, is placed into the category of 'game' or transaction.

Secondly, TA is attractive because it deals with normalcy. For being OK means that one is judged by peers as acceptable to them. TA appeals precisely by staying away from the extremes of experience, and by unifying participants with the consensus of the middle ground. Its energy is directed to promoting an ideal of normality, and developing means for getting people to rapidly identify themselves with it. Many therapies make use of the appeal to normalcy, but TA succeeds, as it puts so many back into the fold of OK-ness.

Berne's innovation was to use the theory of TA directly in the clinical setting. That is why it is commonly called 'educational'. The special terms – P-A-C, OKs, strokes, etc. – are taught in the first session and serve to define what ensues. Theory and practice collapse into each other. Hence it is a highly practical theory, close to everyday events, and an equally theoretical practice, with everyone analysing everything: 'She's hooked your parent', 'Now you're playing Rapo', 'You just gave out a cold fuzzy' (an insincerely affectionate 'stroke') and so on. Transactional analysis is popular because the theory uses language that is easy to relate to one's own experience. Some interesting consequences follow. In lieu of psychological depth human behaviour turns into a collection of games and ego states, all going around together in the life of the group. The terms are drawn directly from the current consumer society. People now become creatures with 'rackets', who accumulate 'trading stamps' with their neuroses so they can cash in later. They are scripted like characters in a TV situation comedy or game show, playing to the audience.

This therapy involves the direct imposition of a moral standard as the prime instrument of change. The Adult in TA is the element of moral change, and he represents the conventional standards of behaviour. Opposed to the Parent, which is the repository of irrational morality, the Adult is able to stand for good rational morality, backed up by the group. Thus strengthened, the Adult will tame the Child – i.e. the impulses. Morality and the bourgeois ideal are all invoked to stifle the Parent–Child.

Berne and Harris reduce the Freudian triumvirate of id, ego and superego to banal levels on the theatrical stage of real life. To be OK, all anyone has to do is accept adult definitions of reality, and conform to established order. The results are obviously conformist and simplistic but that doesn't automatically stop the process being therapeutic.

TA has the virtue of being straightforward. And therapies such as TA, which are so potentially conformist, may be directly exploited for political ends. TA is used, for example by business corporations, prisons, and the military for making people get along better. Where human relationships in any context are in some way difficult and ineffective, consideration of the type of transactions involved should provide some answers.

Further reading

Berne, E. (1961). *Transactional Analysis in Psychotherapy*. (New York: Grove Press)
Berne, E. (1964). *Games People Play*. (New York: Grove Press)
Berne, E. (1972). *What do You Say After you Say Hello? The Psychology of Human Destiny*. (New York: Grove Press)
Berne, E. (1976). *Beyond Games & Scripts*. (New York: Grove Press)
Freed, A. (1976). *TA for Teens*. (Sacramento: Jalnar Press)
Freed, A. and Freed, M. (1977). *TA for Kids*. (Sacramento: Jalnar Press)
Harris, T. (1967). *I'm OK - You're OK*. (New York: Harper Row)
Steiner, C. (1974). *Scripts People Live*. (New York: Grove Press)
Woollams, S. and Brown, M. (1979). *The Total Handbook of Transactional Analysis*. (Englewood Cliffs: Prentice Hall)

Section V
SOME ECLECTIC APPROACHES

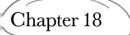

Chapter 18

GROUP THERAPY

The history of group therapy stretches back to the dawn of recorded time. In a sense the early Greek dramas offered a type of psychological release not much different from the psychodrama we will discuss in a moment. Prayer meetings, revivals – even the hypnotic seances that Mesmer conducted in Paris in the late 1700s – are the ancestral forms of today's therapy groups.

Group therapy did not gain any scientific notice, however, until 1905, when a Boston physician named Pratt made a fortunate mistake. Pratt found that patients suffering from tuberculosis were often discouraged and depressed. He first believed their despondency was due to ignorance about the disease they suffered from. So he brought them together in groups to give them lectures about 'healthy living'. The lectures soon turned into very intense discussions among the patients about their problems. Pratt discovered that his patients gained much more strength from learning they were not alone in their suffering than they did from his lectures.

By 1910 group treatment was used by many European psychiatrists who gathered together people with similar psychological problems for 'collective counselling'. Moreno tried group psychodrama in Vienna with displaced persons, children and prostitutes. By 1914 Adler suggested that group techniques might be a more effective way of helping large numbers of clients than the usual one client–one therapist encounters.

Kurt Lewin evolved the Training Group (T-group) technique in 1947 but these developed as a separate stream from group psychotherapy, in teaching institutions where the aim was to facilitate understanding of group processes in normal people, with the object of improving the group functioning in the task-orientated organization from which the individuals came. The staff generally had backgrounds in teaching or social psychology, and there was little interchange at first with the clinical field. The basic feature of the T-group arose more or less by accident when the group members of the original experiment, attended the subsequent staff discussion among the leaders of the groups. The leaders, at first apprehensive at sharing their own responses and thoughts with the members as the latter did with them and each other, found that they had stumbled on an immensely powerful learning situation; this feedback principle was subsequently built into the T-groups themselves.

Increasing exchange has taken place between the T-group and clinical field over the last 10 years, with modification of both. On the clinical side the influence has been towards greater emphasis on openness and frankness, and the confrontation of clients with their 'here and now' interaction in the group, and towards greater willingness of the therapist to express his own responses to group phenomena. On the T-group side, there has been more concern with the individual's response, and in California particularly, T-groups have tended to be seen as 'therapy for normals' – ways of enhancing human potential and experience, and combating the increasing alienation of the individual from his personal and social roots.

Therapists of all the various orientations (psychoanalytic, humanistic and behaviourist) have modified their techniques to be applicable to therapy groups. And group therapy has been used successfully in a wide variety of settings – in hospital wards, with both psychotic and neurotic patients, in outpatient psychiatric clinics, with parents of disturbed children and with delinquents in correctional institutions. Typically, the groups consist of a small number of individuals (6–12 is considered optimal) with similar problems. The therapist generally remains in the background, allowing the members to exchange experiences, comment on one another's behaviour and discuss their own problems as well as those of the other members. Initially the members tend to be defensive and uncomfortable when exposing their weaknesses, but they gradually become more objective about their own behaviour, and more aware of the effect their attitudes and behaviour have on others. They gain an increased ability to identify and empathize with others in the group, and a feeling of self-esteem when they are able to help a fellow member by offering an understanding remark or a meaningful interpretation.

So when we talk about group therapy today, we may mean any psychological treatment that is carried out by a group. We could be referring to analytic therapy, client-centred therapy, Gestalt therapy, T-groups, encounter groups, behaviour therapy or a dozen other varieties of therapy. In other words, the term 'group therapy' no longer conveys very much specific information.

Why conduct therapy in a group? The answer depends partly on the type of therapy in question, but there are two general advantages. First, group treatment obviously represents a more efficient use of the therapist's time, and so it is a good deal cheaper for the clients. Second, certain treatment objectives lend themselves to a group setting, and in fact might be difficult or even impossible to achieve in a one-to-one therapy setting. For instance, if you want to learn how you 'come across' to others, a group setting will clearly be a better choice than individual treatment. A group provides a client with a choice of behavioural models, as well as massive social approval or disapproval for a client's actions. A group can create a sense of belonging that is important for growth. The group may also serve as a mini-society where a client can safely question certain patterns of his or her own behaviour – for instance, is the client typically dominant or submissive in social situations? Clearly, there are potentials in a group that are not available in individual therapy.

Group therapy probably provides the greater part of long-term psychotherapy in the National Health Service in Britain now, in view of the economy of scale.

Although the various forms of group therapy treatment differ considerably among themselves, as you now will be well aware having read about such approaches as Gestalt therapy and Rogerian client-centred therapy, they all appear to be based on the belief that intimate sharing of feelings, ideas, experiences in an atmosphere of mutual respect and understanding enhances self-respect, deepens self-understanding and helps the person live with others. There are six main advantages to the group approach:

(1) The knowlege that other people are in much the 'same boat' can reduce the client's anxiety, and may give the client courage to express his or her deeper feelings.

(2) Listening to others and talking through ideas with them may stimulate the client to recall and relive similar experiences.

(3) Hearing how others have solved their problems may suggest to the client new ways of handling his or her difficulties.

(4) By expressing emotions in the presence of a sympathetic group, the client may dissipate some of the feelings of fear or guilt that are retarding the client's progress.

(5) Acceptance and support by the group may give the client the reward or encouragement needed to put new solutions into practice.

(6) The group may act as a 'social theatre' for the client to try out new ways of behaving before having to use them in larger social settings.

A group in terms of group counselling is characterized by members who 'interact psychologically with purpose in pursuit of a common goal'. Such a group is more than a collection of people because the group members share some common attitudes and values, accept each other and relate to each other in many ways. They accept membership in the group to deal with the problems they have in common as well as to satisfy some individual needs, and the desire for membership ensures that they conform, at least minimally, to the group standards. Mahler (1969) has defined group counselling as a social experience that deals with developmental problems and attitudes of the individuals. It is the process of using group interaction to facilitate deeper self-understanding and self-acceptance. There is a need for a climate of mutual respect and acceptance so that individuals can loosen their defences sufficiently to explore both the meaning of behaviour and new ways of behaving. The concerns and problems encountered are centred in the pathological blocks and distortions of reality.

Group counselling may be preventative and/or remedial for the person involved. Preventative counselling for the individual permits him to resolve concerns prior to serious problems developing, while for those individuals who have developed more serious problems, group counselling can be a process of intervention to change behaviour. The group may be more powerful than a counsellor in individual counselling as power is exercised in two directions. Firstly, the group is made up of peer members, and the feedback from the peers regarding the self has been seen as more potent and more important to the member than that of a single counsellor. The group feedback can also give consensus regarding perceptions of the individual's behaviour, and this consensus from the group will be more powerful than the person's self insight or the feedback from the counsellor. Additionally, the group can also exert power against the counsellor in an attempt to protect the individual, so the individual will feel more secure in a group of peers than he would in meeting the counsellor in a one to one relationship. In this way the group can provide an element of security.

WHY GROUP COUNSELLING?

The rationale for group counselling seems deeply rooted in the nature of human beings and their societal relationships. Personality is to a certain extent the product of interaction with other significant human beings, and the need of people to be closely related with others is seen as basic as any biological need and essential to their survival. People desire to be liked and accepted but they differ in their degree of sociability, hence some seek out and belong to more groups than others and some participate more than others in the groups to which they belong. The usefulness of the counselling group is that it becomes a microcosm of society where the members and the leader can observe patterns of behaviour and then work through those 'problems' that need to be resolved. These 'problems' are usually based to some extent on a social interaction and are, therefore, best solved or resolved in a social setting, the group.

Mahler (1969) usefully sets forth statements describing situations in which individual counselling should be utilized, and the appropriate conditions for group counselling. The following are composite lists containing some of Mahler's indications:

Individual counselling indicated for:	Group counselling indicated for:
(1) Crisis situations complicated by a quest for causes and possible solutions	(1) Individuals who need to develop a more positive self concept
(2) Situations in which confidentiality is needed to protect client and others	(2) Individuals who need to learn deeper respect for others, particularly those who are different, and to learn to share with others
(3) Interpretation of test data	(3) Persons who need to gain social skills (talking and relating to others) and overcome interpersonal problems
(4) Individuals who exhibit extreme fear of talking in a group	(4) Individuals who are able to talk about concerns, problems, values and find peer support helpful
(5) Persons who are so grossly ineffective in relating to peers that they may not be accepted by group members	(5) Individuals who need others' reaction to their problems and concerns
(6) Situations in which extremely deviant sexual behaviour is involved	(6) Individuals who prefer to involve themselves slowly in counselling, and who can withdraw if it becomes threatening

(7) Individuals who have a compulsive need for attention and recognition

(7) Those who feel a lack of purpose and direction in their lives or ineffective in controlling their lives i.e. coping with stress

(8) Severely depressed persons who are too withdrawn to participate in a group

(8) Those who have poor academic study, work or marital performances

(9) Paranoid personalities who are overly distrustful and suspicious of the group members

(9) Persons who have difficulty in expressing or controlling their feelings such as love or anger, dependency and assertiveness.

(10) Schizophrenics who are too disturbed in their thinking and out of contact with reality at times

(11) Alcoholics and drug dependent persons who tend not to stick to long-term commitments. Such persons benefit more from highly structured groups of similar clients after individual therapy and cure, e.g. AA.

(12) Hypochondriacs and narcissistic persons both in their own ways alienate themselves in a group, since they wish to focus entirely on themselves.

There is some agreement among therapists about the desirable characteristics needed in the potential group member: (1) He is motivated: he wants to change, is prepared to work for it and his wish to enter the group is entirely voluntary. (2) He has a particular expectational set: he has a high opinion of group therapy and does not view it as second rate or inferior to individual therapy; he believes that the group will suit his needs and prove beneficial. (3) He has sufficient psychological and verbal sophistication. Shertzer and Stone (1976) and Mahler (1969) among others, all indicate the psychological significance of group membership, for adolescents in particular. As adolescents grow their emotional needs urge them to seek a variety of social experiences and interests, and group participation can enable adolescents to develop the capacity for mutual interpersonal interaction. The group offers a great range of momentary and continuing experiences that enable its members to grow and develop.

Given a conducive environment the individual can risk lowering his defences and can begin to explore areas that are normally threatening. The individual may feel that his problems are unique, but in feeling free to bring these problems to the group that person often finds others have experienced the same or similar problems. In the sharing of common problems and feelings, alternatives can be discussed and methods formulated to change the situation so that the individual can cope more effectively with it. The atmosphere of the group should convey a sense of understanding, sensitivity and assistance, which will promote self worth in that no matter what the individual does, or says, he can be accepted and cared for. However, the individual in this situation develops a responsibility to self, in that the individual is free to identify his unique concerns and to make decisions about whether to focus on them or not.

Characteristics of group counselling primarily reveal that it is a thera-peutic experience for clients who do not have a serious emotional problem. As Mahler (1969) points out we should not expect group counselling to change deep-seated emotional and neurotic problems. The major goals appear to be concerned with helping normal people and less seriously neurotic persons recognize their problems and solve them before they become serious. In general terms group work focusses on social, emotional and self concept development.

ORGANIZATION OF GROUP COUNSELLING

The group needs clear expectations, a real purpose, effective leadership, meaningful participation, the necessary security to enable members to openly contribute their ideas and reactions, and the ability to commun-icate with each other. The counsellor functions as a leader but functions within the group. His chief job is to help the group establish a friendly atmosphere in which members can explore problems and relationships. Empathy, respect, genuineness and concreteness are the claimed characteristics the counsellor must have towards his clients if any goals or objectives of group counselling are to be achieved. Although these facili-tative conditions have been noted in relation to the counsellor it becomes paramount that group members offer the same conditions to each other, and members must accept each other. The counsellor serves as a model in providing an atmosphere that is safe enough for self-exploration.

Should a group be balanced in a particular way or should it admit a range of clients assessed as likely to benefit from therapy? There is no clear answer to this issue. Homogeneous groups, consisting of clients with similar problems, e.g. alcoholics, drug addicts, homosexuals and over-weight people are relatively easy to form as they have basically similar goals for all their members. Heterogeneous groups, typical of long-term therapy, contain clients with a variety of problems; they need a diverse 'social world' to learn about themselves and others and to try out new forms of behaviour. The group should be so constituted that opportunities for learning are optimal. For instance, a group consisting only of passive-dependent members will permit minimal scope for learning alternative ways of relating. Similarly, a unisex group will be rather limited in helping a patient with heterosexual difficulties! If group members are too homogeneous, members merely support one another's basic inter-personal orientation to such a degree that alternative perceptions in ways of behaving, which are needed for optimum change and growth, are not provided.

When age and sex are not the determining factors in selection of members, attention must be given to similarities in background and personality. If too many differences in these areas exist, the problems of communication may be so great that the group may be unable to function. One area in which a difference in background seriously affects the group's functioning is a discrepancy in verbalization ability.

It has been argued that single sex groupings are preferable on the basis that in a mixed group where a masculine model of competence prevails women who follow the stereotypical role of dependence, submissiveness and receptiveness are reinforced for that behaviour. But other experienced counsellors generally advocate single sex groups for younger students, but see an advantage in mixed groups for adults particularly where such areas as social skills and heterosexual difficulties are involved, on the theory that full socialization depends upon being comfortable and skilled in dealing with both sexes.

Having selected suitable clients the counsellor must determine the size of the group. With children small groups of 4–6 are the norm. For adolescents the group functions best with 6–8 members and an optimum number of 10 with adults. As groups increase in size, transference reactions become weaker and weaker until members experience no meaningful relationships with each other. Most therapists conclude that 4–8 is ideal for group counselling; it is a natural grouping – the largest group that can function without a leader and some strong rules – and larger groups would break up without strong leadership. In order to reap the full benefits of group counselling, clients must be able to accept considerable responsibility for themselves and function as a group. A group fewer than 5, however, is likely to be ineffective because the range of behaviour patterns is too narrow and the pressure on each person to participate is too great. With more than 10 members some may not get adequate attention and others can avoid involvement. When the group is too small it ceases to operate as a group, and the individuals find themselves involved in individual counselling within the group setting. In addition, opportunities for utilizing the dynamics within the group are reduced, and pressure may be put on the individual so that he cannot choose to remain silent, and the comfort level is reduced. The upper limit is determined by the fact that less time is available for working through individual problems when there are additional members.

The results of numerous studies indicate a marked reduction in interactions between members when the group size reached 9 members, and a second marked reduction when it reached 17 or more members. Mahler (1969) commented that groups of 20 plus require more leader direction and may resemble an educational experience more than a counselling experience. He acknowledges that it is possible to develop a good working climate in a large group but the group will probably be orientated toward personal exploration and understanding of human behaviour rather than toward deep involvement and a commitment to changing behaviour.

Closed group versus open group is also a consideration. A closed group is one formed with a specific number of counsellees, and thereafter no new individuals are brought into the group. The open group is flexible with changing membership, where a core of counsellors with some experience in an ongoing group work with new arrivals as others depart. An old member may terminate and someone new is selected by the group or the counsellor. Dinkmeyer and Muro (1971) suggest that closed groups are preferable. Primarily a group must develop, it must move or pass through certain phases for optimal effectiveness. Such movement requires time, continual interaction and a sense of cohesiveness. Closed groups give more security and stability for the group to develop along the suggested lines. A closed group is effective in that it has a stable population and time limits within which to work, whereas the open group members may be more aware of the transitory nature of their relationship.

In an open group the number of meetings could vary for each member but in a closed group it is possible to specify a number of meetings. The advantage of a specific number of meetings is that a time limit on the life of the group is provided and members are forced to work within that span. Shlien, Mosak, and Dreikurs (1962) found that the imposition of a time limit on the life of a group aided the determination of the group to reach specific goals and tended to eliminate aimless discussion. Although some intensive groups meet 2–5 times a week, the majority of groups meet once a week. Mahler (1969) suggests a minimum of ten sessions for most group counselling but obviously the life of the group will be determined by the nature of the material to be explored, and by the developmental stage reached when termination has been envisaged. It may be necessary to renegotiate the duration time of the group with the members. It has been found that counselling may be more effective if groups terminate after a designated period and perhaps reopen at a future date. Presumably members may have time to consider topics which have been discussed or pursue various suggestions for problem solving, and then after several weeks when the group meets again further discussion may ensue.

However, if the counsellor is informed by the group that they have discussed all that they want to for the present then the counsellor should structure for closure. Two to five sessions are recommended for closure. During these tapering off sessions, the counsellor should assist members of the group to summarize, clarify and restate the problem areas that have been covered.

The sessions, *per se,* may last an hour if they take place once per week, 2–3 hours if meetings take place every other week. Sessions less than 35 minutes do not allow the group to approach and develop topics, whereas sessions longer than 45 minutes result in boredom. The suggestion of 2–3 hours would, therefore, seem too lengthy. Probably the time factor may depend on the age of group members or initially how familiar members are with each other or even the topics under discussion.

STAGES OF GROUP COUNSELLING

Group counselling progresses through four stages. Most researchers would agree on this although each researcher uses a different terminology. The first stage Mahler (1969) terms 'the involvement stage', Dinkmeyer and Muro (1971), the pseudo group. During this first stage the counsellor should clarify the purposes for meeting, encourage members to get acquainted and share hopes, goals and expectations with the beginning of a trusting, acception relationship between members and between members and counsellors. It is a difficult stage punctuated by awkward pauses, hesitant statements and polite talk. Initial sessions of counselling tend to be superficial and non-group orientated. Individuals have no sense of 'we-ness' or groupness and other members though physically present do not represent important individuals in his life. The group leader is the central figure and the target of any group hostility. Many topics are touched on fleetingly in these early meetings with no real depth of discussion.

The transition stage represents movement from an essentially social atmosphere to a therapeutic–educational atmosphere. Structuring is now required, and the leader should concentrate on encouraging individuals to share their feelings. The real structuring is done by the way the counsellor functions within the group – knowingly or unknowingly encouraging certain behaviours and discouraging others. The completion of the transition stage is indicated by a rather clear commitment (not necessarily verbal) to utilize the group for one's own learning.

Following this is the working stage, characterized by a high morale level and a definite feeling of belonging. The individual comes to realize that the group is part his. Principles are aimed at helping the member change any ineffective behaviours and attitudes. Group counsellors may utilize the group interaction to increase understanding and acceptance of values and goals and to learn and/or unlearn certain attitudes and behaviours. The counsellors' task is difficult; it is an art of knowing when to make a suggestion, provide information, when and how to challenge clients to action and when to support clients' efforts to face disturbing feelings. At this point in group life there is open and direct communication. A creative use of ideas is now possible and leader dependency is minimal. Individuals receive both positive and negative feedback and member-to-member confrontation is common.

The final stage or ending state is gradual. As was pointed out earlier 2–5 sessions may be needed. A feeling of rejection on the part of the members is almost inevitable when the group is ending.

EVALUATION

Much of the research work which has been conducted into group counselling has suffered from methodological deficiency. Many studies have tried to evaluate the effects of group counselling on individuals without an adequate comparison with individuals who have not received the treatment. Without control it is impossible to evaluate unambiguously the effects of an independent variable such as group counselling, and consequently many studies have been criticized for failing to use control groups. Some studies have used control groups but have been criticized because they have been conducted over too short a period of time, using immediate rather than long-term criterion measures. Group counselling is not a method for obtaining rapid change, and the criteria – the goals and objectives – involve such personality variables as increased self-acceptance, being more effective in interpersonal relationships and better problem solving which are long range objectives and cannot be expected to result from a short series of meetings. Hanley (1971) in investigating the effects of short-term group counselling upon the measured concerns and level of anxiety of students found that in the non-counselled control group, concerns and anxiety level significantly increased. In the short-term counselled group (6 sessions) concerns and anxiety remained relatively stable, while in the longer-term counselled group (12 sessions) concerns and anxiety decreased in number. These results suggest that positive group counselling outcomes are improved by increased number of contacts. Truax (1968) and Luria (1959) and most other therapists, all found that group counselling improved self concept, but without an agreed definition of self it is difficult to make an evaluation of improvement.

Group therapy offers the client access to interpersonal neurotic patterns. We get to see ourselves as others see us. While the therapist can help the individual with some of these problems, the final test lies in how well the person can apply the attitudes and responses learned in therapy to relationships in everyday life. This points out the advantage of group therapy, in which clients can work out their problems in the presence of others, observing how other people react to their behaviour and trying out new methods of responding when old ones prove unsatisfactory, e.g. peer relations or authority conflict problems. These experiences are difficult to duplicate in a one to one setting. The group is a microcosm of society and provides realistic and lifelike social situations useful for modifying social habits, attitudes and judgements of group members.

Opportunity for free expressions of opinions and emotions with a less personal reference is available within the group counselling situation. Members of the group very often realize that their concerns, their problems etc. are not idiosyncratic. It is often a relief to clients to find other peers who feel as they themselves do; it eliminates the feeling of being 'odd one out'. Individuals come to a fuller realization and acceptance of self and others during discussions. Whilst this is not achieved by all members, many may gain an increase in self-confidence, an improvement in social skills and a reduction in tensions. Getting several people's reactions to one's problems and concerns does tend to put everything into a proper perspective. Mutual acceptance, affection, respect and helpfulness within the group tend to develop improved self-concepts. In addition group therapy commends itself in a contemporary period of economic retrenchment as it makes more effective use of scarce resources. Therapist time, therapist/client ratios, through-put of clients are all positive recommendations, but only if the clients involved in such an approach are suitable. Client–therapy match must remain the sole criterion not economic viability.

What then, are the limitations of group counselling? Most researchers feel that whilst confidentiality is essential it is difficult to achieve. It may be difficult in individual counselling particularly if the problem is a legal or moral one, but in group counselling it is even more difficult to expect clients to keep secret another's innermost problems. However, this must be a 'rule' which all members must accept before committing themselves to group counselling.

In the group counselling situation, there may be less warmth or closeness of relationship between the counsellor and individual group members. Some may need to identify more directly with one person before being able to relate or interact comfortably with a group.

The counsellor has less control of a group than an individual. Tasks of the counsellor are also more complicated in group counselling. He has to understand the speaker's feelings and help the speaker become aware of them but also must observe how the speaker's comments influence other group members. Helping clients in groups, therefore, requires careful study and understanding of the process of interpersonal behaviour.

A group approach may in fact be slower and less efficient than the individual approach, as most group members may wish to contribute some idea in a discussion this takes time. Personal problems of a particular member may become secondary to the more general problems of the group or to those of another member. The counsellor must try to ensure that problems of all students are dealt with. Group treatment cannot go as far or deep into a person's life as can individual therapy. The reason is not simply dilution of attention by the other members.

But overall, provided suitable clients are chosen, participation in group counselling can help people learn to be more natural, less defensive, more open to the richness of feelings, with an increasingly deeper capacity to enjoy living and experiencing.

Further reading

Bennett, M. E. (1963). *Guidance & Counseling Groups*. (New York: McGraw-Hill)

Dinkmeyer, D. and Muro, J. (1971). *Group Counseling: Theory & Practice*. (New York: Peacock)

Kaplan, H. and Sadock, B. (eds.) (1971). *Comprehensive Group Psychotherapy*. (Baltimore: Williams & Wilkins)

Kreeger, L. (ed.) (1975). *The Large Group*. (London: Constable)

Mahler, C. A. (1969). *Group Counseling in Schools*. (Boston: Houghton Mifflin Co.)

Napier, R. and Gershenfeld, M. K. (1973). *Groups: Theory & Experience*. (Boston: Houghton Mifflin)

Ohlsen, M. M. (1970). *Group Counseling*. (New York: Holt, Rinehart & Winston)

Rosenbaum, M. and Berger, M. (eds.) (1975) *Group Psychotherapy & Group Function*. (New York: Basic Books)

Schertzer, B. and Stone, S. (1976). *Fundamentals of Guidance. 3rd Edn*. (Boston: Houghton Mifflin)

Thompson, S. and Kahn, J. (1970). *Group Process as a Helping Technique*. (Oxford: Pergamon)

Walton, H. (ed.) (1971). *Small Group Psychotherapy*. (Harmondsworth: Penguin)

Yalom, I. D. (1975). *The Theory & Practice of Group Psychotherapy*. (New York: Basic Books)

Chapter 19

FAMILY AND MARITAL THERAPY

Over the last decade these therapies have become popular and fashionable practices, particularly among behaviourally oriented therapists and social work counsellors. It is not another type of therapy but essentially a redefinition of the therapeutic task itself. The therapy may involve a variety of the approaches already considered, but whichever is employed the focus of the therapy is the family or the marriage rather than the individual.

FAMILY THERAPY

Family therapy is a logical and obvious device for treating much of the emotional and social distress clients report for two reasons. Firstly, everyone is a member of this primary group even if their contacts at times are tenuous. Secondly, within the family are contained the most intimate and strongest emotional and social experiences of our lives. All this suggests that many neuroses and antisocial behaviours have their roots in disturbed family relationships. Therapeutic intervention at the family level should, therefore, benefit individual members of the family. Therapists were quick to discover that the problems of a troubled child are often embedded in pathological interactions within the family. Even if the therapist were able to help the child in individual psychotherapy, the child would have to return to a family life that supported old, inappropriate ways of behaving. In these cases therapists with family orientations quickly moved away from working with the identified client to working with the whole family to facilitate changed ways of interacting.

Although it had long been customary in British Child Guidance Clinics for a mother to be interviewed as well as her child, she was usually seen by a social worker while the child was interviewed and treated separately by a psychiatrist. Ackerman (1966) first began using family interviews in work with children in the USA. This is being increasingly practised in Britain, where some child psychiatry clinics have been re-named departments of child and family psychiatry. Family therapy can be seen as a natural development of child psychiatry. Skynner (1976) is a leading exponent of family and marital therapy in Britain. As you will have realized, the therapies discussed so far in this book treat the individual *qua* individual and apparently ignore changes that may be necessary in the environment outside the treatment room. Yet the client spends a majority of his life within the family setting, a setting which may undo all the work the therapist has been trying to achieve. Neither is the family really affected by what happens in the individual therapy.

Family therapy takes on an ecological philosophy, a systems analysis of the pattern of relationships in which family members live. What comes to the fore in family therapy is reality, not the fantasy of Gestalt psychodrama, or of the psychoanalytic transference process. The father, mother and sibling rivals are truly there, joining in sharing, clarifying and expressing from their own perspectives.

Family therapy groups include one or even two therapists (usually one male and one female), the client and the client's immediate family. The family group may consist of husband and wife or of parents and children. On the assumption that the individual's problems reflect a more general maladjustment of the family, the therapy is directed toward helping the family members clarify and express their feelings about one another, develop greater mutual understanding, work out more effective ways of relating to one another and solving their common problems. Sometimes family therapists will conduct their interviews in the family home, particularly when they work on the crisis intervention model.

Although some family therapists concentrate their therapeutic work on the most responsive family members, others may involve associated networks too, such as workplace and neighbourhood (Speck and Attneave, 1973). However, most limit themselves to the nuclear family, perhaps with key grandparents or with others sharing the home.

Members of a family or a marital pair must accept that the problem they seek help with is a shared one and have a joint responsibility in its solution. To establish a therapeutic alliance, which has to include family members as well as therapists, there needs to be some residual mutual goodwill, and a wish for things to improve.

How co-operative spouses or leading members of the family are, how willing they are to help and share in taking responsibility for the problems and their resolution, is itself of diagnostic importance; for example a continuing attempt to make one person the repository of all disturbance or blame suggests that the other members need to see and keep it that way.

Liberman (1970) has noted three crucial aspects in the application of therapy in the family context.

(1) Creating and maintaining a positive therapeutic relationship. Since we are dealing with the whole family unit the relationship, concern and empathy must be with *all* members of the family, both as individuals and as part of the family system. The therapist should reinforce and model the harmonious and rewarding aspects of family life so that these are strengthened through his words, actions and attitudes.

(2) Making a behavioural analysis of problems. The therapist's first goal is to determine what each family member sees as the problems within the family and what each hopes to achieve through family therapy. The therapist tries to determine how the problem that is presented relates to the family network and how the family maintains a homeostatic balance among members. Family rules are uncovered. Some rules are overt – such as those that state when bedtime is, and who is supposed to cut the grass – and some are covert – such as 'Don't take your problems to sis. She is too mixed up'. The family may make a scapegoat of one family member (often the identified client) as having all the problems in the family. The therapist, in collaboration with the family, will seek answers to two major questions.

   (a) What behaviour is maladaptive or problematic – what behaviour should be increased or decreased? Each person is asked:
      (a) What changes would you like to see in others of the family?
      (b) How would you like to be different from the way you are now?
      The answers enable the therapist to choose carefully specific behavioural goals.

   (b) What is maintaining undesirable behaviour or reducing the likelihood of more adaptive responses? The mutual patterns of social reinforcement in the family must be scrutinized in this analysis, since their deciphering becomes central to an understanding of the case and to the formation of therapeutic strategy. Often a teenager's unacceptable behaviour, for example, is being maintained by inconsistent management: Dad says she should be in by 10 pm but Mum stays up and lets her in quietly at 12 am whenever Dad is on night-shift; a primary school child learns with astonishing skill to play off one parent against another; a toddler manages effectively to break up a marriage by screaming unless his mother always sleeps in his bed rather than with her husband. When what is happening is understood in terms of what is being reinforced, then the specific behavioural goals, together with how they can be achieved, often become infinitely clearer. The next step is to alter the reinforcement condition.

(3) Deciding on and implementing a therapeutic programme, the family therapist will try to (1) improve communication within the family, (2) encourage autonomy and empathy among family members, (3) help the family develop new ways of making decisions, and (4) facilitate conflict resolution.

Sometimes videotape recordings are used to make the family members aware of how they interact with each other. Parents with a problem child may be taught to observe carefully their own and their child's behaviour to determine how their reactions may be reinforcing certain responses and extinguishing others. For example, a child's temper tantrums and abusive behaviour may be inadvertently reinforced by the attention they elicit. The counsellor may often draw up what amounts to a contract, i.e. a series of small-scale goals which the members of the family can agree to reach, and to help each other to reach, together.

It is vital that the earliest small-scale goals should be easily attainable, so that members of the family readily achieve them, and thereby not only enjoy the satisfaction of doing so but are reinforced to attempt the more difficult goals in the series by their earlier success. For example, it might be important for success or failure to avoid a goal such as 'Dad to take more interest in the children, and the children to help more in the house' in favour of simpler and specific activities. For example, for a given week the goals might be:

(1) children wash up dishes after the evening meal and make their beds every morning,
(2) Dad takes the children to a football match on Saturday afternoon to give Mum some peace and quiet,
(3) Mum tidies herself up for Dad when he comes in from work.

In this specimen week each family member is involved in a bargain or contract which has the effect of rewarding another or other members of the family by changing his own behaviour; but in return each member of the family is also rewarded by the changes in the behaviour of the others. Such a written form of the weekly contract, signed by all the family (devised by the counsellor in discussion with the family) helps maintain involvement, and acts as an index of what has already been achieved when things become difficult at later stages.

The role of the therapist is both to enable the family to achieve small but regular success in attaining the small-scale goals which are established from week to week, by limiting the objectives of each weekly contract so as to be reasonably sure that they can be achieved, and to offer encouragement and reinforcement as small gains are made.

As Liberman writes, these tactics can be conceptualized as 'behavioural change experiments'. Liberman (1970) describes a behavioural approach to family therapy in the case of Mrs D., a 35 year-old housewife and mother of three, who had a 15 year history of severe headaches. Hospital investigations had found no organic reason, and 18 months of intensive, psychodynamically oriented psychotherapy had provided no relief; her practice had, therefore, been to stay in bed for several days at a time. On those occasions her husband would become very solicitous and concerned, giving her a great deal of attention. In his behavioural analysis of this relationship, the therapist gently explained the role which Mrs D.'s headaches were playing: only when Mrs D. was ill did she receive the reward of her husband's attention; it was, therefore, to her advantage, as she perceived it, to become ill frequently. The therapist was able to form a close, non-critical and supportive relationship with both members of this partnership and gradually, by keeping a detailed record of their occurrence, to show them the pattern which existed between periods of illness experienced by Mrs D. and her husband's gratifying changes in behaviour.

Liberman reports that through a close and trusting relationship with both partners, he was able to teach the husband how to be more demonstrative to and appreciative of his wife on a day-to-day basis, so that he took a deeper interest in the management of the children and his wife's activities in general. Similarly, he was able to teach the wife how to be responsive to her husband's efforts, to tell him how she liked his inquiring about the events of the day, and how much she enjoyed the evening outings they began to make together. Liberman goes on:

> Mr D. was instructed to pay minimal attention to his wife's headaches. He was reassured that in so doing he would be helping her decrease their frequence and severity. He was no longer to give her tablets, cater to her when she was ill, or call the doctor for her. If she got a headache, she was to help herself and he was to carry on with his regular routine insofar as possible. I emphasised that he should not, overall, decrease his attentiveness to his wife, but rather change the timing and the direction of his attentiveness.

Within ten sessions, both were seriously immersed in this new approach toward each other. Their marriage was different and more satisfying to both. Their sex life improved. Their children were better behaved as they quickly learned to apply the same reinforcement principles in reacting to the children.

It is reported that a year later a follow-up call to Mr and Mrs D. found them continuing to progress.

Family therapy has been found useful in treating schozophrenia where, for the hapless individual, the handling of everyday reality is so difficult. Many psychotic patients are found in families whose members cannot individuate themselves from each other. Laing implicates family pathology in the aetiology of schizophrenia (see Chapter 20). Some psychiatrists (Laing, 1964; Bateson, 1956) believe that the immediate family of schizophrenics may be at least as ill as the patient. They are thought to communicate in deviant ways such as 'double binding' the patient by presenting to him contradictory overt and covert requirements to which there is no correct response and from which there is no escape; for example, the mother who repeatedly asks her son to kiss her, but moves away when he comes towards her, and then accuses him of not being a good son. Such families may have disturbed styles of thinking and illogicality which conceal underlying hostility. A schizophrenic reaction in this situation becomes a natural self-protective response (Laing and Esterson, 1964). In consequence, schizophrenia is seen by some as a family problem, and family therapy, therefore, as appropriate in certain cases.

While family conflicts are not generally seen as having a primary role in the aetiology of schizophrenia, it is well-established (Brown, Birley, and Wing, 1972) that patients who have had a schizophrenic breakdown are more liable to relapse in an emotionally charged family atmosphere. So for some, the family is not the place to be, and one outcome of family therapy may be a decision to split up for the benefit of all concerned.

Family therapists are increasingly finding that disturbed patterns also help produce physical ailments, from asthma to heart attacks and – some are convinced – even cancer. Dr Salvador Minuchin, Director of the Philadelphia Child Guidance Center, has aleady attracted wide attention with his work on anorexia nervosa, the 'starvation disease' . . . Now Minuchin and his team are concentrating on asthma and diabetes. In one case of diabetic sisters, ages 12 and 17, doctors found a metabolic defect, but only the younger sister responded to drugs and diet changes. A therapist found out why: each parent constantly tried to get her support in fights with the other parent. The allegiance of the 12 year-old was not sought. Once the parents stopped trapping the older sister in their struggles, she too began responding to treatment.

In many cases, family therapists argue, an outbreak of physical illness is both a symptom of high stress among family members and an attempt to cope with it. Minuchin says that anorexia nervosa victims are 'saviours of the family' because they paper over parental conflicts that threaten to destroy the family. Philip Guerin, Director of the Center for Family Learning in New Rochelle, NY, finds that many fathers suffer heart attacks shortly after a grown son or daughter leaves home. His hypothesis: the child may have functioned as a buffer for parental conflict.

So family therapy has abandoned the usual one to one isolated relationship of traditional therapy to take on the client's whole family, with the aim of exposing and breaking family patterns that create emotional and physical disorders in individual members.

One advantage of family therapy is that it tends to be relatively less expensive and briefer than individual treatment. It also enables a person to focus more directly on the real behaviours that affect life with those closest to him. Certain aspects of the emotional world that appear right away in family treatment may remain unnoticed to any form of individual therapy. In addition, family therapy allows for a more comprehensive approach to other kinds of environmental problems besides the interpersonal. Family treatment tends to promote more responsible attitudes towards other people, in contrast to individual therapies whose emphasis on the self may pass over into selfishness. Family therapists argue that very genuine individual growth can be achieved under their treatment. 'The promotion of a more mature mode of relationship within the family offers a definite version of a rather universally held vision of emotional well-being within our society – that of individual freedom coexisting with interdependence.' (Kovel, 1976 p. 259)

Family therapy would seem to be the best recourse in marital difficulties, alcoholism and adolescent disturbances. In all these situations, the problems arise from or come to infect the whole family unit, particularly where economic and physical disadvantage also lie in the background.

MARITAL THERAPY

The number of people seeking help for their marital problems has increased enormously. There were 715 000 divorces in the United States in 1972, and it has been estimated that 40 million American married couples need counselling. In Britain there has also been a steep rise in petitions for divorce – over 146 000 in 1976, from 28 000 in 1960.

Since the end of the Second World War, there have been large scale social and psychological changes which have had a profound effect on the expectations and behaviour of couples and families. Thus the greater level of equality sought and obtained by women and the scientific control over procreation has had a major impact on the man–woman relationship.

As material standards have risen, expectations have increased for fulfilment at the next layer of being, that is to say for emotional and instinctual fulfilment (Dominian, 1972). Men and women now expect – consciously and unconsciously – far more from each other and are less prepared to tolerate lower standards of personal happiness.

Factors contributing to marital dissatisfaction emanate from several sources. At the most elementary level the pressure of material needs and the presence of gross and cruel behaviour in one or both spouses are relevant whilst, at a more advanced level, more subtle emotional factors play a part. In a study of 600 couples seeking divorce with children under the age of 14, Levinger (1966) noted that in general, middle-class spouses were more concerned with emotional and psychological factors, whereas lower socio-economic class spouses were concerned with financial stability and the absence of physical aggression in their partners.

Dominian (1972) has produced a model of the marital life cycle and suggests three phases during which any of five areas of relationships between a couple can become disturbed, though some areas are more prominent at one phase of the marital cycle than another. In Dominian's model there are five main relationships between a couple: physical, emotional, social, intellectual and spiritual. The therapist, instead of relying on his intuitive grasp of the 'marital problem', will find it useful to analyse the complex range of material the couple offers him in terms of the five relationships by noting in which of them the most important difficulties occur. Thus, if a sexual (the physical relationship) problem is central, the therapist can readily determine whether this problem exists alone or whether it is a manifestation of, or co-exists with, disturbance in any of the other four relationships. Such a differentiation serves as a guide to treatment. Thus, for example, if the sexual relationship alone is disturbed, the therapeutic approach is likely to be a behavioural sex therapy, such as that described by Masters and Johnson (1970). If, on the other hand, the emotional relationship is also impaired and this seems the chief problem, the couple will be helped with this, before their sexual difficulties are tackled.

Marriage has a life cycle of its own too in Dominian's model, divisible into three phases: the first phase comprising the first five years, which brings the couple to their late 20s or early 30s on average; the middle phase, covering the period during which the children are growing, and ending about the late 40s or early 50s when the youngest child has left home; and the third phase when the marital partners return to the state of being a couple and ending with the death of one of them. This division is helpful as certain problems are phase-specific or more likely to take place during one phase than another. Thus problems that occur during the third phase are unlikely to be present in the two preceding ones.

In assessing marital pathology, the therapist can place the couple in the appropriate phase and note which of the five relationships are disturbed. A brief outline of Dominian's phases follows.

First phase

Physical relationship

Sexual problems, if present, are relatively uncomplicated in that they do not result, usually, from emotional difficulties but spring directly from poor technique and lack of knowledge and so respond well to sex therapy.

Emotional relationship

Some relationships seem to evaporate emotionally within the first marriage year. A close examination of the background of such a marriage shows that the husband or wife or both were not really ready to commit themselves to a permanent relationship with all that this implies; often there has been uncertainty about their own identity which has not been resolved by further growth but by negotiating a social event, namely a marriage. This has given them a status before society but has not resolved their confusion. As the weeks and months pass they continue to behave as if they were single people, unable to narrow their relationship to each other. They find each other increasingly distant and strange and have little in common, so much so that they gradually realize that they married for reasons such as the need to escape from home, loneliness or status seeking.

Uncertainty of commitment to the relationship may result when one or both partners have trouble disengaging from their parents. This common problem may be reinforced by the inability of the parents to let go and a collusion is forged – the parents hold onto the child. Where a mother has tried to dominate and retain the male child, hostility is likely to show in his behaviour to the new wife. His hostility may be acted out by returning late regularly from work, using offensive language, getting drunk or having an affair. This behaviour is intended to demonstrate that no woman is going to rule his life. Even when detachment from parents does occur, a danger still exists that one partner may treat the other as a parental substitute. In the case of both partners seeing the other as a parental figure, they tend to idolize each other and have difficulty coping with hostile or ambivalent feelings. The relationship is inevitably unstable.

In some marriages there is a fierce independence, in which the husband, usually, is battling with his fears of being submerged, exploited or lost in the world of women. This independence may be associated with excessive participation in manly pursuits, defiance and stubbornness against any exhibition of dependence on women, and usually an aloofness from any overt display of tenderness and intimacy.

The arrival of a baby can be a threat to a husband. He may seek comfort by having an affair, or be unable to visit his wife at the hospital or ignore the arrival of the child. The baby may consume all the wife's attention and lead temporarily to her losing interest in the outside world and in her husband. She may become depressed although in most cases this is short-lived.

Social relationship

In some spouses (husbands in particular) a combination of factors lead to excessive drinking, gambling or in passing a great deal of time away from home with a resultant disturbance in the social relationship.

Intellectual and spiritual relationship

Sometimes a marriage is entered into hurriedly without the partners' awareness of each other's intellectual abilities and interests or value and moral system. After a short while when the couple realize that they have little in common in these spheres their relationship is threatened and may well peter out.

Second phase

All the problems of the first phase discussed above may occur in the middle years. There are, however, according to Dominian, some features unique to the second phase.

Physical relationship

No particular sexual problems occur in this phase apart from the wife's loss of interest in sex following the birth of her children, and increased dis-satisfaction in either partner with sex that has never been satisfactory but it was hoped would improve with time.

Emotional relationship

With the passage of time – as the couple gradually acquire more self-confidence and feel more differentiated in terms of their identity – their relationship inevitably changes. If one partner of an interdependent pair becomes more resilient, the security of the other is threatened. When a previously dependent wife, for example, grows more self-confident she may begin to insist on conducting activities formerly carried out by her husband: using the car, having her own set of friends, collaborating on financial decisions and the like. Couples usually change together, but if the wife's change is unilateral and the husband opposes it, she may increasingly feel her freedom and independence curtailed. Initially conflict is emotional; later, as it escalates, the wife may show her anger by withdrawing from sex and finally, if the husband is unco-operative she may seek an alternative relationship. In the latter part of the second phase, either partner may face the crisis of 'middle-age'. For example, the husband may find that although he has reached a certain peak in his career he has not achieved his own private goals; the wife on entering her menopause may perceive it as the end of her femininity and sexuality (Dominian, 1972). This is also a time when the children, now usually late adolescents, contribute problems of their own – their need for independence for instance – which commonly have an effect on the parents' marriage. Marital therapy may need to be replaced by a family approach.

Social, intellectual, and spiritual relationship

Sometimes the social relationship may change because one partner has moved into a different social milieu leaving his spouse behind in the original setting whence they both came; this leads to conflict and ultimately to possible marital rupture.

Third phase

Sexual relationship

A problem may arise if there is a decline of interest in sex in one or other partner. Until the work of Masters and Johnson (1970), there had been a widely-held misconception that sexual interest and performance waned after middle-age, particularly in women. This misconception still lingers and can lead to difficulties in the sexual relationship.

Emotional relationship

The process of change that began in the second phase may continue into the third. This sometimes underlies the painful experience of a middle-aged wife whose husband has an affair or leaves her for a younger woman. There may be several reasons for the husband's behaviour, including his need to ward off middle-age sexual identity anxieties, or his attempt to enjoy the freedom and range of activity – appropriate to a man of his twenties – at a much later age when self-confidence and ego differentiation make it possible.

Social, intellectual and spiritual relationship

Change over the years may leave a couple distant from one another as they discover that their values, and social and intellectual interests have drifted off in different directions. If there is a marital problem, the therapist will want to see both partners. He will take pains to invite the co-operation of the other members of the family (or the spouse), and if possible interview them together. This conjoint interview is often conducted by a pair of therapists, male and female, which is particularly useful in marital therapy, as it avoids some of the dangers of appearing to take sides. Ideal marital therapy is conducted with both partners together. This immediately raises a possible problem: one spouse may refuse to participate. Whatever the reasons, every effort should be made to persuade the missing partner to attend at least once, and for them to be seen preferably together as a couple.

Basically the therapist plays active roles as facilitator and teacher, and through his words and actions aims to change the couple so that they can perceive the nature of their marital difficulties and learn new modes of relating towards one another. The couple, in the course of treatment, should perceive the way they see each other (that is the projections they place on each other), the power structure in their relationship, their manner of communication – both verbal and non-verbal, and the areas in which the minimum needs of each is not being met by the other. All this can be accomplished by the therapist's interpretations and, more importantly, by the way he outlines in an exaggerated way the couple's pattern of relating, particularly their methods of communication.

The marital therapist will also draw the attention of the couple to the type of non-verbal communication between them: an expression of anger, eyes raised to the ceiling, a vacant look, clenched fists, swinging of the legs, a sarcastic smile, nodding of the head; all these convey a wealth of feeling and significance of which the partners have hitherto been unaware. Within the framework of a trusting, safe relationship with the therapist, channels of communication develop and these in turn facilitate the expression of a wide range of feelings, many of which have been suppressed for months or years. Hopefully, there is a clarification of problems and recognition of mutual needs and responsibility.

Examining the pattern of power in the marriage is another common task for the therapist. In a relationship in which the sharing of power has failed, endless battles are waged over who is boss. In these circumstances, the wife in particular complains that her husband makes demands on her without respecting her wishes and treats her as if she were a servant. The therapist plays a useful role in clarifying, with the couple, the pattern of the conflict for power; his objectives are that they recognize the nature of the conflict and develop respect for each other's separatedness and autonomy. What is often missing in disturbed marriages is the expression of tenderness and affection.

While marital therapy, like family therapy, is somewhat eclectic in approach, an emphasis on behavioural rather than psycho-dynamic principles appears to have greater pay-off. This is because such treatment is more simple and is suited to most couples who want to deal directly with their problems and not plumb the depths of the dynamic factors that underlie those problems (Stuart, 1969).

In adopting a more behavioural line, the therapist makes a careful case history of the presenting problems. He then assesses both areas of conflict and areas of satisfaction in the marriage in order to set up a hierarchy of the needs of each partner. The husband may, for example, want more sex or forgiveness and understanding for an extra-marital affair. The wife may want greater time spent together at home or more tenderness in love-making or more open communication. The principle underlying this approach is that both partners give to the other something they need or want and receive something in return. It is a contract which, as in family therapy, as it is fulfilled will bring more fulfilment of the expectations, needs and understandings of both – reinforcing future interaction along the same lines. For example the husband may agree not to go out drinking with his friends more than once a week and help more with the housework; in return his wife will allow him to have a beer each evening at home and will no longer need to punish his evening absences by sexual withdrawal.

As in family therapy, where the therapist has to ensure that no one member becomes the collective bearer of the family's difficulties – the scapegoat – so in treating a couple great care needs to be taken not to label one partner as sick and more in need of help than the other. The therapist emphasizes from the outset that the problem to be tackled is the relationship between the couple not either member of it.

If the initial interviews engage the family or couple, they may continue to communicate more openly between sessions, particularly as they come to recognize their mutual responsibility for change. This is one of the clear advantages of conjoint therapy: participants go on living together between sessions, and so have an opportunity to put into practice new ways of interacting begun in the sessions and to make the mutual change for the better. When they slip back into the old maladaptive ways, they may point this out to each other; in other words they can continue as their own therapists. For this reason, family and marital therapy sessions are often held at less frequent intervals than those in individual therapy, or group therapy with strangers. Ideally, the couple should be seen together at intervals of between one and four weeks. The frequency is dictated by the following factors. If the couple have manifold and complex problems which need to be clarified and understood before any progress can be made, intervals should be weekly or bi-weekly. Similar frequencies are indicated when anger and hostility are so marked that incessant rows simply poison the therapeutic atmosphere, and in the case of spouses who both have particular personal needs which require the therapist's active intervention. Once the couple have sufficient awareness of their problems or the hostility has abated or their individual needs have been met, intervals between sessions can be increased. In effective marital therapy, the couple should achieve some new insights and more effective coping mechanisms in each session; they then need time to apply what they have learnt to the marriage and discover '*in vivo*' what changes occur. After this is accomplished, the frequency of sessions can be reduced to monthly or six-weekly.

Therapy terminates in a variety of ways: one spouse refuses to continue and the other sees no point in coming either; both partners are happy with the outcome and suggest termination – this is accepted by the therapist or he recommends additional interviews to confirm their sense of optimism; the therapist takes the initiative and indicates that no further therapy is required, or that there is little purpose in continuing at this stage.

Sexual dysfunction

The 1970s have seen a remarkable increase both in the availability of treatment for sexual problems and in the demand for it. Masters and Johnson (1970) have pioneered this development, most of the current forms of 'new sex therapy' being derived from their approach. Their methods have been pragmatic, not based on any school or theoretical model of psychotherapy or behaviour change.

The category of sexual dysfunction traditionally covers such problems as erectile failure, premature or delayed ejaculation, and the inability of the woman to experience orgasm or to become sexually aroused. Whilst these 'target–organ responses' are a fundamental part of the problem it is important to deal with them in the context of a sexual relationship, or, for the individual, the sexual self-image. As yet, a satisfactory classificatory system which incorporates both the physiological, and the psychological and inter-personal aspects has not been devised.

The goals of sex therapy can be broadly defined as follows:

(1) Helping the individual to accept and feel comfortable with his or her own sexuality
(2) Helping the individual to initiate and maintain sexual relationships
(3) Helping the couple to improve the quality of their sexual relationships.

Often problems under (1) have to be faced when dealing with (2) and (3), whereas (2) assumes that no stable relationship exists. Sex therapy is a good example of 'behavioural psychotherapy', the principles of which are as follows:

(1) Clearly defined and appropriate behavioural goals are set and the client asked to attempt to achieve them before the next session.
(2) Those attempts and any difficulties encountered are examined in detail.
(3) The attitudes, feelings and resistances that make those behavioural goals difficult to achieve are identified.
(4) Those attitudes, etc are modified so that achievement of the behavioural goals becomes possible.
(5) The next behavioural goals are set, and so on.

A basic feature of this approach is that the client or couple always has something to do between treatment sessions. Usually these tasks are small steps towards the final goals, though they may involve keeping records or otherwise monitoring behaviour as part of the analysis necessary for treatment.

In Skinnerian terms, behaviour is being shaped by successive approximations to the desired objective. The therapist may devise a finely graded hierarchy of situations, beginning with something the patient can behaviourally manage and proceeding all the way up to the target symptom. For example, a sexually frightened couple might be instructed not to do anything more erotic than simply lie close to each other the first week; remove articles of clothing the second week; kiss on the lips the third week; fondle bodily parts the fourth week; and so on and so on, until the two are so desperate and eager that they could achieve their mutual requirements without any likelihood of failure on a crowded London bus. In this sort of sequencing, there is also an inbuilt systematic desensitization as the couple face and overcome at each stage a previously challenging, or repulsive or threatening scene in the sexual script.

Throughout the whole of the sex therapy the responsibility for change lies with the couple or individual. Constructive use must be made of the help of the therapist. The latter can do little unless the clients are prepared to attempt the behavioural tasks recommended for their 'homework'. However, the therapist must ensure that the clients do have the time and opportunity to carry out the tasks. It can be that treatment is deliberately delayed by the therapist until a house move, job change or relative's visit is over before the therapy commences free of distraction.

Sex therapy varies in duration but on average requires about 12 sessions spread over 4 or 5 months. This is in contrast with the concentrated daily sessions of the 2 week programme advocated by Masters and Johnson (1970). The more intensive format is impracticable within a non-private setting where usually once-a-week sessions are the most frequent that can be practically arranged. Research experience with a 'correspondence course format', in which the couple were seen on only three occasions over 4 months, corresponding weekly in-between (Mathews, Bancroft, Whitehead, Hackman, Julier, Bancroft, Gath and Shaw, 1976), and a comparison of weekly and monthly counselling regimes over a similar period (Carney, Bancroft, and Mathews, 1978) indicate that some couples may do better with less frequent sessions. Autonomy and self-confidence is perhaps enhanced by the reduced dependence on the therapist.

Further reading

Bancroft, J. (1974). *Deviant Sexual Behaviour*. (London: Oxford University Press)
Beels, C. and Ferber, A. (1969). Family Therapy. *Fam. Process*, **8**, 280
Block, D. A. (1973). *Techniques of Family Therapy*. (New York: Grune & Stratton)
Erickson, G. and Hogan, F. (1972). *Family Therapy*. (Monterey: Brooks Cole)
Glick I. D. and Kessler, D. R. *Marital & Family Therapy*. (New York: Grune & Stratton)
Kaplan, H. (1975). *The New Sex Therapy*. (London: Baillière Tindall)
Masters, W. and Johnson, V. (1970). *Human Sexual Inadequacy*. (London: Churchill)
Minuchin, S. (1974). *Families & Family Therapy*. (London: Tavistock)
Skynner, A. C. (1976). *One Flesh, Separate Persons*. (London: Constable)

Chapter 20

SOCIAL AND ENVIRONMENTAL THERAPY

INTRODUCTION

Up until fairly recently most of our laws, customs and philosophies have been based on the assumption that mental illness existed entirely within an individual. Most forms of therapy can be seen as attempts to cure the client by working on him alone.

Within the last 30 years rather a different point of view has emerged – a belief that mental illness is as much a disruption of relationships between people as it is a disruption of one person's inner psychodynamics. Abnormal behaviour is almost always expressed in social situations – unless 'crazy people' disturb or upset others, they are seldom sent to mental hospitals or to see a therapist. Treatment must not merely alter the functioning of the client's body or brain, or change his personality – it must also help the client reorient him or herself in society. Indeed, in many instances, the group of people around the client may actually be contributing to the 'craziness' without realizing it. In such cases the best form of therapy may be removing the person from that environment – or somehow getting other people to behave differently toward the client.

There has developed a realization of how sensitive we all are to our environments. The ecologists have demonstrated rather vividly the disasters that may occur when we pollute the physical world around us. But man does not die from lead poisoning alone – polluted psychological environments can kill or corrupt a man's spirit as readily as dirty air and contaminated water can kill or corrupt his body. The job of the environmental psychotherapist is similar to that of the ecologist – to identify the sources of psychological pollution and remove them. For example, a hospital is as dependent on the social system in the institution as the rest of

237

us are dependent on plants and rainwater. From a psychological point of view, some hospitals are barren deserts that 'starve' their patients of intellectual and emotional stimulation without meaning to do so. Through our study of the biological aspects of ecological systems, we are learning how to make deserts blossom. Perhaps someday we will learn similar psychological techniques for making institutions such as mental hospitals 'bloom'.

APPROACHES AND PRINCIPLES

In social and environmental therapy there is an over-riding concern with the social milieu in which the client resides, and how such an environment may inhibit or may be used to facilitate recovery. The terms social therapy, and environmental therapy do not lend themselves to precise definition, and other terms have also been employed to describe this general orientation towards treatment, e.g. milieu therapy, community therapy and social psychiatry.

Austin suggested that social therapy refers to the attainment of treatment goals by the use of techniques designed to positively influence various factors in the environment, and the effective use of social resources.

Social therapy, environmental therapy, milieu therapy, community and social psychiatry will be, despite variations in approaches and emphases, taken as synonymous in this introductory text since they all appear to be imbued with the following principles of supplying care and treatment.

(1) A recognition that the environment including the hospital, the family and the sub-culture are important determinants of how deviant behaviour is expressed; how it is formally and informally handled, and these factors must be taken into account, and used in any therapeutic intervention.

(2) A properly conceived mental health service will be based on the recognition that both the hospital therapist, a comprehensive range of local authority facilities and family are inter-dependent parts of a total service serving the same population.

(3) Hospital client status in a psychiatric establishment has dangers. The social system of the hospital will influence the norms of the client groups. These norms must be consistent with progress towards self-realization and independence. It is so easy for 'institutional neurosis' to develop.

This institutional neurosis is characterized by extreme apathy, deterioration in personal habits, a humble posture and shuffling gait. The symptoms disappear if the client is encouraged to become more active and is given more contact with the outside world. But even in a modern residential hospital, with an enthusiastic staff and active methods of occupational treatment and group psychotherapy, the client is insulated from the normal tensions of living in his family and working in the outside community, and he may well become dependent on the protected environment of the institution. This militates against improvement. The danger of dependency is much less for outpatients attending day individual and group sessions.

The simplest form of environmental therapy is perhaps the vacation: getting away from it all can often give a person a fresh perspective. Psychiatric social workers show their awareness of this fact when they recommend removing a child from an unhealthy family situation and putting the child in a foster home. Helping mental clients find jobs and comfortable living quarters outside the hospital is another form of environmental therapy practised by social workers. Rehabilitation centres often teach disturbed people how to function better in work situations, how to relax, how to play or paint or read or make music, how to meet people and stay out of trouble with the law – all ways of helping people make healthier adjustments to presently-existing environments.

If the therapist cannot easily find ways of removing the 'psycho-pollution' from the client's world, or of helping the client live more happily despite the pollution, then more radical treatment is usually needed. Typically this takes the form of moving the client to different surroundings – such as a mental hospital. Once we called such places 'asylums' – safe, comfortable places to which a client could flee when the storms of life became too threatening. Unfortunately, mental hospitals all too often became rubbish dumps, huge edifices crammed with human rejects. As ecological systems such hospitals were often more destructive to human functioning than was the outside world the clients had sought relief from.

Social/behavioural therapists tend to see mental illness as being caused by unhealthy living conditions. The best form of treatment, from this vantage point, would surely be putting the client in a new environment or social milieu – each aspect of which would be carefully designed to help the client learn better habits of adjustment.

Many leading psychiatrists came to the conclusion that the hospital itself was a sick organization, with a sick social structure that could not make a positive contribution to help its sick clients. It became increasingly apparent that only by transforming the organization and by exploiting its total therapeutic potential could it make a distinctive contribution to helping the whole person. Such a view required exchanging the concept of cure and emphasizing the need for re-socialization and encouraging social competence, in order that the client may take his place in the community to which he belongs.

The British psychiatrist Maxwell Jones is an exponent and initiator of such an approach, establishing a 'therapeutic community' concept in what has been termed 'milieu therapy'. In a hospital therapeutic community the customary clinical hierarchy has been exchanged for client participation, and executive control is in the hands of a multidisciplinary team, answerable to the community as a whole – clients and staff.

Writing in the *American Handbook of Psychiatry* in 1959, Dr Louis Linn points out that our concept of therapy has changed over the years:

> In former days there was a tendency to regard treatment in the mental hospital as that which takes place during the fraction of a second when the current flows from an electro-shock apparatus, or during the longer intervals involved in other therapies . . . In the therapeutic community the whole of the time which the patient spends in the hospital is thought of as treatment time, and everything that happens to the patient is part of the treatment programme.

Viewed in this way, Linn continues, the trees and flowers on the hospital grounds and the decorations in the wards, the way the food is served and the behaviour of all hospital personnel – without exception – are part of the treatment programme.

Though it does not replace other forms of treatment, milieu therapy does attempt to make the total environment a 'school for living' in which the client can develop new attitudes and build more rewarding social relationships. In a sense the therapeutic community is rather like a non-stop 24 hour-a-day encounter group. However, its primary function is not usually that of removing symptoms or merely changing behaviours; its aim is said to be that of drawing the client into normal relationships that will give the person confidence, self-esteem and social competence.

The Maxwell Jones type of therapeutic community in a residential hospital is usually a fairly small unit with face-to-face gatherings of all members, social analysis of events, opening of communications, flattening of the authority pyramid and blurring of roles. It is composed of both staff and clients with both groups expected to relate, for therapeutic purposes, to the maximum degree possible, rather than to individual therapists. This is less immediately gratifying to many clients and therapists than individual treatment, but may ultimately help the clients more, if they are able to become mature enough to relate to the larger group.

A standard feature of the community is a daily meeting of staff and clients. Common recurrent themes for discussion are rejection, violence, sexuality, dependence and independence, staff friction and relations with outside bodies.

The essence of social therapy is openness of communication and shared examination of problems. Clients are encouraged to use their initiative in running their own lives. They learn that they have an active role to play in helping themselves and each other, by participating in communal life. The possibilities are open to them of discovering the personal and inter-personal problems that may have been troubling them. They can learn to express themselves openly, particularly their feelings towards themselves and others, as well as learning social skills and attitudes. The Group meetings play an important part in facilitating these processes. Social therapy is seen as being particularly useful for helping the neurotic and psychotic client who does not function socially, perhaps never did, whose condition may require long-term care, and where short-term psycho-logical therapy either has been exhausted, or is inapplicable. In short, the focus is on social functioning rather than on psychopathology. The therapist will be concerned with influencing groups, social organizations, community networks rather than persons seen in isolation one from another.

With some schizophrenics, Brown *et al.* (1972) and Laing (1964) have urged that they be removed from the family home and placed in a more therapeutic community, since a family in which there is high emotional expressiveness seems to provide a detrimental social environment for a schizophrenic. Despite this view many therapists now regard the family as a major supportive structure in the social therapy strategy. As we noted in Chapter 19, counselling will often be helpful both to the relatives, and indirectly to the client. One aim of such supportive psychotherapy is the transfer of some of the source of support from professionals to a client's family. This task if often no easy matter. Caring for a neurotic of psychotic relative calls for perseverance and discretion. For the family to be successfully incorporated into supportive therapy however, requires that they be properly informed and counselled. They need to be instructed as to what to do and how to do it. In addition the family needs help in their own right in caring for their ill relative as the process can be extremely burdensome at times.

It is too early to evaluate the long-term effectiveness of social therapy, though short-term effects appear to be beneficial in terms of social development, self-esteem and self management. However, it is unrealistic to assume that such techniques and therapeutic communities could be developed in all hospitals and therapy settings, for it requires staff who are committed to the concept, who are willing to throw off their status and roles and involve themselves as equals in an ethos of self questioning and change. The therapeutic milieu is lively and creative, but also stressful and confronting.

Not everyone, staff or clients, is comfortable in this atmosphere, though many adjust and learn to value it. The question of whether some may find it anti-therapeutic is still open to research. One of the disadvantages of social therapy is that it is difficult for a client to opt out, if it does not suit him in the form provided in a particular unit, except by leaving or not co-operating.

Having markedly changed the social organization of hospitals in order to try and reverse the effects of institutionalization, serious questions are now being raised about the merits of admitting clients to hospital without compelling reasons for so doing. Hospital client status is accorded to an individual who has been selected for this role by others, i.e. members of his family, general practitioner or other medical and social agencies. However, some important questions ought to be raised with the neurotic and psychotic, e.g. what can be achieved by hospitalization that could not be obtained by the client remaining at home? Are there any disadvantages to admission – in a particular case – that might outweigh the benefits? Will reinforcement of the sick role by admission to hospital adversely affect the client's eventual re-establishment in the community? etc.

The difficulty in evaluating milieu therapy is the same as with other forms of group therapy – terms like 'confidence' and 'self-esteem' refer to intrapsychic traits, and hence are hard to define or measure objectively. Therapeutic communities certainly are far more humane forms of treatment than the old-style mental hospitals.

Further reading

Clark, D. (1977). The therapeutic community. *Br. J. Psychiatry*, **131**, 553–64

Edelson, M. (1970). *Sociotherapy & Psychotherapy*. (Chicago: University Chicago Press)

Freeman, H. and Farndale, J. (eds.) (1967). *New Aspects of the Mental Health Service*. (Oxford: Pergamon)

Goffman, E. (1961). *Asylums*. (Harmondsworth: Penguin)

Hinshelwood, R. and Manning, M. (ed.) (1979). *Therapeutic Communities*. (London: Routledge & Kegan Paul)

Jones, M. (1968). *Social Psychiatry in Practice*. (Harmondsworth: Penguin)

Lewiz, J. and Lewis M. (1977). *Community Counseling*. (New York: John Wiley)

Section VI
SOME ISSUES IN EVALUATION

Sheri

Chapter 21

EFFECTIVE PSYCHOTHERAPIES OR EFFECTIVE THERAPISTS?

With such a lavish menu of psychotherapy and counselling available, one may well ponder, 'Which method is best?' or 'Who can help me with my problem?' These questions are not easy to answer. Research into the effectiveness of psychotherapy is hampered by several major difficulties. First and foremost is 'How do we define "success"?' Another vital issue is how do we know which treatment variables were responsible? What about the 'placebo effect'? Does each therapy function best with certain types of problems, with particular types of client, with specific therapist personality traits, etc? These and many other problems which permeate the issue of the relative effectiveness of particular therapies have not been resolved as yet.

PROBLEMS IN EVALUATING SUCCESS

Many factors make it difficult to evaluate the effectiveness of psycho-therapy scientifically. Science requires objective events, things that can be readily measured. But by its very nature, most therapy concerns itself with changes that involve a person's thoughts, beliefs and attitudes – elusive changes that can seldom be seen or scrutinized or measured in an objective way. Only Behavioural approaches provide limited and clear-cut measurable goal behaviours, which are either achieved or not.

How do we know that an individual is helped by therapy? We cannot always depend on the client's statement. At the beginning of therapy, many clients may exaggerate their unhappiness and problems, as if to convince the therapist that they are really in need of help. At the end of a course of therapy, they may report feeling better, either to express appreciation to the therapist or to convince themselves that their own expectations were met, and that time and in some cases money were not wasted. These phenomena must always be considered when evaluating the client's view of progress.

The therapist's evaluation of the treatment as 'successful' cannot be taken as an objective criterion either. The therapist has a vested interest in proclaiming that the client is better. In any case, the changes that the person shows during the therapy session may not carry over into real-life situations. Some psychoanalysts evaluate their treatment almost solely in terms of the amount of insight the patient gains about his or her own 'hang-ups' and the changes that occur in the client's basic personality. Since the analyst is the only person who has worked through these problems with the patient, the analyst may consider that he is the only person qualified to judge whether a 'cure' has taken place. The fact that the analyst could not objectively demonstrate to independent observers that the patient was, in fact, 'improved' might be of little importance to such a therapist. Although this position has its merits, other therapists, e.g. behaviour modifiers, offer more objective measures of improvement – such as modifications in the client's overt behaviour and the removal of neurotic symptoms. These changes can be observed and possibly agreed upon by people other than the therapist himself. For example, performing more effectively on the job, able to talk to the opposite sex, drinking less and so on – are more valid, but even these can be difficult to obtain and measure, often requiring long-term follow-up.

Some insoluble difficulties arise in comparing therapy methods, for certain objectives can only be attained by the appropriate method and by no other. For example, it is not possible to carry out a comparative evaluation of the effectiveness of psychotherapy and behaviour therapy in bringing about psychodynamic growth, or greater insight into one's unconscious mental life, and so on. Nor is it possible to compare the effectiveness of behavioural methods of helping retarded children care for themselves with a psychoanalytic approach to that objective. The latter does not address itself to that sort of issue, nor can we decry it for not doing so any more than we can criticize behavioural approaches for not dealing with unconscious processes in the previous example.

If we take an analyst's subjective impressions as our guide, then psychoanalysis would seem to lead to 'full recovery' in 35–40 per cent of the clients, with an additional 15–20 per cent of the clients showing noticeable improvement. If we apply the more objective measure of 'symptom removal', we find that the improvement rate is much lower – 30 per cent or less.

In the humanistic therapies the client usually determines whether the therapy was successful or not. Rogers has developed self concept measures that chart changes in the client's perceptions of his or her progress, but the validity of using the client's subjective impressions as an index of improvement remains in some doubt. The claimed 'cure rate' (client reported) for humanistic therapy is usually in the neighbourhood of 75 per cent or so.

TREATMENT VARIABLES

We can rarely be certain, either, that the therapy has caused the observed changes in a client's behaviour since other variables such as improved physical health, the removal of financial worry, job promotion, examination success, family reunion and the like may have been the real trigger. Even client expectation for improvement rather than the therapy have been shown to be a possible cause of the reduction of phobias (Kazdin and Wilcoxon, 1976). Furthermore, no two therapists who use the same method have the same personality, and no two clients bring the same attitudes, problems and methods of coping with their difficulties to the therapeutic session. Therapist variables and patient variables interact inextricably with treatment methods, making it difficult to assess which factors are related to a successful outcome. Experienced therapists tend to be more effective than inexperienced therapists, though, whatever the type of therapy involved (Garfield and Bergin, 1978).

To complicate the picture still further, some people improve if they think they are receiving effective treatment (the placebo effect). And a sizeable number of people, both psychotic and neurotic, will get better without any treatment – spontaneous remission! The rate of spontaneous remission must be used as a baseline for evaluating any form of therapy, as we shall see shortly in considering Eysenck's criticisms of the effectiveness of psychoanalysis. Despite these difficulties, a number of controlled studies indicate that (1) psychotherapy does help, and that (2) different therapeutic approaches do not differ greatly in effectiveness (Smith and Glass, 1977).

The question that concerns most current researchers is not 'Which therapeutic approach is best?' but rather, 'Which method is most effective for a particular problem?' The latter question is difficult to investigate because it requires finding a large number of people with the same degree of the same problem and assigning them randomly to different treatment conditions; as we have seen, behaviour disorders differ markedly from one person to the next. Current opinion indicates that some of the behaviour therapy techniques are more effective in treating specific anxieties and phobias than is either psychoanalytic or client-centred therapy. The conclusions of Luborsky *et al.* (1975) on the comparative success of various therapies was that psychosomatic symptoms are treated more successfully by psychotherapy plus medical regimen than by medical regimen alone; and second behaviour therapy is especially suited to treatment of 'circumscribed phobias', specific compulsions and sexual problems.

EYSENCK'S ATTACK ON THE EFFECTIVENESS OF PSYCHOTHERAPY

Behaviourist psychologists in particular have levelled strong criticisms against the 'unscientific ways' in which the effectiveness of psychotherapy is usually determined. After the Second World War, Eysenck investigated several thousand cases of mentally disturbed servicemen and women in British hospitals. He reported in 1952 that the overall improvement rate among those clients given psychoanalytic treatment was about 44 per cent. The improvement rate for clients given any other form of psychotherapy was about 64 per cent. Several hundred other clients received no psychotherapy at all; their physical ailments were treated as necessary, but they were given no psychological therapy. The spontaneous recovery rate for the untreated neurotics was such that about 45 per cent of them recovered within a year of the onset of their illness. By the end of the second year, this figure rose to 70 per cent; and within 5 years about 90 per cent of all untreated cases were either dramatically improved or 'cured'. Although we must always keep in mind what we mean by the term 'cured', it does seem as if the effectiveness of any form of psychotherapy must be measured against Eysenck's figures on spontaneous recovery.

Eysenck (1952), therefore, argued that there was no justification for the belief that psychotherapy had any beneficial results. If a very high proportion of people with so-called neurotic symptoms get better without any treatment at all, psychotherapy, in order to justify itself, must improve upon this spontaneous remission rate.

This serious challenge to psychotherapy produced a flurry of research, learned papers, claims and counterclaims. The psychoanalysts responded that Eysenck's criteria for improvement were considerably different from their own, since he focused on easy-to-measure behaviour changes. Eysenck ignored all of the basic alterations in the client's personality that are the stated goal of most psychoanalytic treatment. The analysts also raised the important issue of client selection. Some clients are better suited for analysis than others, and the usual feeling is that hospitalized psychotics make the worst clients of all. De Sharmes, Levy and Wertheimer (1954) and Sanford (1954) criticized Eysenck's conclusions on the basis of his having included questionable data, and indiscriminately pooled data from reports with differing criteria for treatment and improvement. Eysenck replied with another paper, 'The effects of psychotherapy: a reply', in 1955.

Eysenck's claims have had a positive benefit, in that they stimulated a considerable amount of research aimed at disentangling the plethora of variables which interact in the treatment context; this, in the long-run, can only be of benefit to the clients of the future. A number of studies are of relevant interest in the 'effectiveness' debate.

The 1953 APA study

In 1953 the American Psychoanalytic Association undertook its own survey of all the people undergoing analytic treatment in the entire United States. Although data were completed on some 3000 patients by the end of 1954, the analysts could not agree among themselves as to what constituted success. When the results of the APA study were finally published in the late 1960s, the only figures reported were for 'symptom removal' – a disappointingly low 27 per cent. Many well-known psychoanalysts reject the APA study as not coming to grips with the intrapsychic changes that do occur during therapy.

Cambridge-Somerville Youth Study, 1953

Teuber and Powers compared 325 potentially delinquent boys who received supportive counselling or psychotherapy with 325 untreated boys who formed a control group. Over a 10 year period the researchers found no overall average differences between the two groups in terms of what had been previously agreed would indicate improvement.

Temple University Study, 1975

Sloane and his colleagues in Philadelphia selected 94 patients suffering from moderately severe neuroses and personality disorders who had come to an out-patient clinic for help. Roughly one-third of the patients were treated with a brief form of psychoanalytic 'insight' therapy; another third received behaviour therapy; the rest were told that they would have to wait at least 4 months for help and acted as an untreated control group. Each client was interviewed before treatment to determine how disturbed he was and what symptoms he showed. The client was also given several personality tests, including the MMPI. Close friends or relatives of the client were also interviewed to get this person's evaluation of what might be troubling the client. After the intake interview, the client was randomly assigned to one of the three groups mentioned above. The assessing psychiatrists did not perform the therapy themselves; they merely evaluated the clients before and after treatment.

Clients in the treated groups were given an average of one hour of therapy a week for 4 months. Clients in the untreated control group were contacted every few weeks to find out how they were doing, and were encouraged to 'hang tight' until a therapist could see them (these calls, of course, were themselves a type of treatment). At the end of 4 months, all the untreated clients who still wished for help were put into therapy. At the end of the 4 month period, the client was again interviewed by the assessing psychiatrist, who did not know (and was told not to ask) what kind of therapy (if any) the client had been given. The client retook the personality tests, and the close friend or relative was seen again to determine what progress this person thought the client had made. Psychiatric assessments of the clients were also made 1 year and 2 years after the experiment began.

Sloane and his associates measured as many different aspects of the therapeutic situation as they could. Some of the tests or assessments they employed were objective, and were aimed at determining success in symptom removal, bettering job performance, improving relationships with others and so forth. Some of the measures were subjective, having to do with how well the client liked the therapist (and vice versa), the client's inner feelings about his or her improvement, the amount of anxiety the client was experiencing, the perceptions that the interviewing psychiatrist and the client's friend or relative had about changes in the client's emotions and behaviours, and so forth. In addition to these rather specific measures, the assessing psychiatrist, the client, the friend or relative and the client's therapist (in two of the groups), also made what Sloane calls 'global evaluations' of the amount of improvement shown by the client. The results of this study can be summarized as follows:

(1) Some 80 per cent of the clients given either behaviour therapy or psychoanalytic treatment showed significant symptom removal, but so did 48 per cent of the clients in the no-therapy control group. Thus either type of therapy is better than nothing, but spontaneous recovery did occur in about half the untreated clients.

(2) Since Freud believed that anxiety is the hallmark of neurosis, psychoanalysts typically hold that the reduction of anxiety is a sign of improvement. Both the treated groups showed a significant reduction

in anxiety, but the no-therapy clients also improved so much that Sloane and his colleagues conclude that the difference among the groups were not really significant.

(3) A frequent complaint made by neurotic clients is that they have trouble keeping a job or in making progress in their careers. At the end of 4 months of treatment, the behaviour therapy clients showed significantly greater improvement in their work situations than did the psychoanalytic or the no-therapy clients. The latter two groups of clients performed about the same.

(4) As far as social adjustment was concerned, the behaviour therapy and the no-treatment clients showed significant improvement. Those individuals given psychoanalytic therapy did not do as well.

(5) The 'global evaluations' of client improvement yielded the most marked differences among raters. As judged by the assessing psychiatrists (all of whom had psychoanalytic training), 93 per cent of the behaviour therapy clients showed improvement, while from the client's point of view, only 77 per cent of those in the behaviour therapy group, 81 per cent of those in psychoanalytic treatment, and only 44 per cent of those in the no-therapy group felt they had improved. It would seem that those clients denied therapy believed they couldn't possibly have got much better without treatment, despite the objective evidence to the contrary noted by the assessing psychiatrists.

We can surmise, in explanation of these findings, that the clients in the two treatment groups probably had quite different notions of what improvement ought to be. Psychoanalysis is an insight therapy, the goal of which is usually to give the person better understanding of his or her mental processes. Behaviour therapy is a broader-scale type of treatment, in which self-help and self-improvement in many areas are emphasized. It is possible that psychoanalytic clients did notice a marked improvement in their mental processes and, believing this to be the major goal of therapy, rated themselves highly. The assessing psychiatrists, knowing that things like good job performance and healthy social relations are also necessary to survival, downgraded the insight clients because they had in fact shown little improvement in these areas (while the behaviour therapy clients had).

(6) Additional findings by Sloane and his group were equally interesting. You may recall (Chapter 10) that one of the major objections raised against behaviour therapy was that it merely removed symptoms without curing the underlying cause of the neurosis, hence other symptoms would develop to replace those the therapy had done away

with. However, Sloane and his associates found no evidence for symptom substitution in any of the clients in any group. On the contrary, it seemed that when a client's primary symptoms showed improvement, the client often spontaneously reported improvement of other minor difficulties as well. Another objection brought against behavioural treatment is that it is a 'cold and mechanistic way of pushing people around'. In fact, the clients in behavioural treatment rated their therapists as being significantly 'warmer, more involved, more genuine, and as having greater and more accurate empathy' than the insight clients rated their therapists as being.

Psychologists have known for years that any therapist does better with some types of clients than with others. Sloane and his colleagues found that their psychoanalytically-oriented therapists did better with well-educated, middle- or upper-class, verbally fluent clients than with relatively uneducated or verbally passive clients. The behaviour therapists did about as well with one type of person as with any other. Perhaps for this reason, none of the clients given behaviour therapy got worse, while one or two people in the other two groups showed a marked deterioration over the 4 month period.

Data gathered 1 and 2 years after therapy had begun tended to confirm the findings made at the end of the initial 4 months. However, direct comparisons were difficult to make for many clients had dropped out of therapy or had disappeared, and all of the 'no therapy' clients were put into psychoanalytically-oriented therapy rather than into behaviour therapy.

Sloane and his colleagues conclude that behaviour therapy is at least as effective as, and possibly more so than, psychotherapy with the sort of moderately severe neuroses and the personality disorders that are typical of clinical populations. This finding should help to dispel the impression that behaviour therapy is useful only with phobias and restricted 'unitary' (simple) problems. In fact, only the behaviour therapy group in this study had improved significantly on both the work and the social measures of general adjustment at 4 months. Behaviour therapy is clearly a generally useful treatment.

One of the most puzzling aspects of the Sloane study is that the analytically-trained therapists saw less improvement in their clients than did the clients themselves or the outside assessors. The behaviour therapists were just the opposite. An explanation of this finding may come from research by Greenspoon (1955), he demonstrated how important the attitude of the therapist is in affecting the behaviour of most clients. Greenspoon noticed that when a client begins talking about sexual abnormalities, or about bizarre thought patterns, the psychoanalyst may unconsciously encourage the client to continue talking. He may lean forward, look very interested, and say to the client, 'Yes, yes, tell me more about that'. But when the client is speaking normally or discussing solutions rather than problems, the psychoanalyst may believe that little or no progress is being made, and hence may occasionally lean back and look uninterested. In Greenspoon's terms, there is always the danger that the therapist may unwittingly reward a client for 'sick talk' and punish him for 'well talk'.

In more humanistic terms, getting the client to concentrate on achieving mental health may be more important than getting the client to understand the causes of his or her mental illness. It is possible that the insight therapists in the Sloane study focused too much on past traumas and not enough on future growth and self-actualization.

The Lieberman, Miles and Yalom (1973) study
Beginning in 1968, these workers recruited 206 Stanford students who wished to participate in encounter groups, and randomly assigned the students to 17 groups led by experienced professionals. The types of therapy involved were sensitivity or T-groups, Gestalt groups, psycho-drama groups, psychoanalytic groups, transactional analysis groups, Rogerian non-directive groups and leaderless groups. Another 69 students, who applied for participation but who could not be accommodated, were used as a control group.

The subjects were evaluated as carefully as possible before the groups began; further evaluations occurred a week or two after the groups ended, and again 6–8 months later. Participants were asked to rate not only the changes they experienced themselves but those they saw in other group members as well. Group leaders also rated the participants, as did close friends of the participants not themselves involved in the group experience. Objective (behavioural or symptom-change) measures were taken as well as subjective (inner-feeling change) measures. The experimenters themselves all had extensive experience working with various types of groups and were, prior to the beginning of the experiment, favourably disposed toward group therapy.

The study offers little scientific evidence that group therapy is of much value. Indeed, it may often be just the opposite. They report that about 8 per cent of the participants were 'casualties' – that is, people who showed evidence of serious psychological harm and whose difficulties could be reasonably attributed to the group experience. About a third of the group members showed positive changes; about a third showed negative changes; and another third seemed unchanged immediately after the therapy. There were few differences among the various types of groups as far as their effectiveness was concerned. By contrast, more than 60 per cent of the control group students who had no therapy reported no change in themselves, while 23 per cent reported a negative change and 27 per cent reported a positive change.

It would appear that the group situations accentuated both positive and negative changes in the participants, but that the overall effect was about the same as if the groups had never been brought together. Immediately after the groups ended, almost 65 per cent of the group members stated that the experience had been a positive one; 6 months later, their enthusiasm dropped by more than 50 per cent.

There are several other aspects of this experiment worthy of note. First, the group leaders reported that they saw some improvement in almost 90 per cent of the members – a rosy view not supported by the rest of the data. When the participants were asked to rate others in their groups, they reported improvement in but 37 per cent of their fellow group members. There was no significant agreement at all among the leaders, the participants, and the participants' friends as to who had changed and in what ways. Particularly distressing were the number of 'casualties' – and the fact that group leaders seemed unaware that any of their group members had suffered so much.

Lieberman, Miles and Yalom conclude that groups are not particularly effective as change agents, but that they can excel at creating instant, brief and intense interpersonal experiences. They state that this chance to learn something about oneself from the open reactions of others is real, important and often available in our society. But they believe that such experiences are not the crucial ones that alter people permanently. They were prompted to conclude that:

> Encounter groups present a clear and evident danger if they are used for radical surgery to produce a new man. The danger is even greater when the leader and the participant share this misconception. If we no longer expect groups to produce magical, lasting change and if we stop seeing them as panaceas, we can regard them as useful, socially sanctioned opportunities for human beings to explore and to express themselves. Then we can begin to work on ways to improve them so that they may make a meaningful contribution toward solving human problems.

As a result of these many disturbing findings on the effectiveness of various forms of therapy, a change of emphasis has taken place, directing research studies away from relating 'outcomes' to specific therapies, and towards teasing out more subtle variables which operate in all therapeutic contexts, such as attempting to delineate what is the most facilitating therapist personality, what is the role of the expectations of client and counsellor which may or may not be shared. It may be more appropriate to ask not what is the most effective therapy, but what sort of therapist is the most effective, whatever his theoretical leaning.

THE EFFECTIVE THERAPIST

The major review of what happens in counselling was Truax and Carkhuff's book, *Towards Effective Counselling and Psychotherapy*. The main theme to emerge in their review of research on psychotherapy and counselling was that the effectiveness of the process depended very much on the personal qualities of the counsellor, and had little to do with the characteristics of the client.

While Truax and Carkhuff (*op cit*) supported Eysenck's (1952) claim, they detected considerable differences between the 'success rates' of individual counsellors, an important subtlety hidden by Eysenck's general criticism. Truax and Carkhuff write:

Eysenck was essentially correct in saying that average counselling and psychotherapy as it is currently practised does not result in average client improvement greater than that observed in clients who receive no special counselling or psychotherapeutic treatment.

However, they continue:

Some other relatively well-controlled studies show that certain counsellors or therapists do produce beneficial effects beyond that observed in equivalent control groups.

Putting together these two bodies of evidence, it logically follows that if psychotherapy has no overall average effect, but that there are valid specific instances where it is indeed effective, then there must also be specific instances in which it is harmful. That is, to achieve this average, if some clients have been helped, then other clients must have been harmed. This suggestion that psychotherapy and counselling can be for better or for worse is the major starting point for present approaches to practice and training.

Truax and Carkhuff analysed the therapy and counselling studies in which beneficial results had occurred. They found that the common element was not the particular therapy but the personality of the counsellor or therapist. This personality, which seemed to produce positive outcomes for clients, was blessed with three clearly defined characteristics:

(1) Non-possessive warmth: the attitude of caring and acceptance conveyed by a friendly and concerned approach to their clients.
(2) Accurate empathy: the capacity to 'feel with' those who seek help, so that clients 'feel understood'. It is a very special type of understanding however. It is not to be confused with sympathy, for sympathy suggests a difference between oneself and the person for whom one feels sympathy. Empathy can be illustrated quite simply by the phrase 'walk in the other man's shoes and if they pinch you feel the hurt'.
(3) Genuineness or authenticity: the conveying of 'realness', of 'being themselves', as distinct from adopting a role or being defensive in their dealings with clients. It involves the capacity to relate honestly to the client, and reveal oneself as one human being to another. This means that there is no place for the false professional front, for this can be spotted and regarded as deceitful by the client immediately. The counsellor should be able to reveal himself as a human being and not indulge in defensive manoeuvres to maintain a position of false security and authority.

This is not the first time that such characteristics have been identified or proposed as essential ingredients in a therapeutic relationship. In Chapter 14 we have already noted the emphasis placed on these by Carl Rogers. Although his terminology is slightly different, there is little doubt that what Rogers termed 'unconditional positive regard' is the same as what Truax and Carkhuff are attempting to convey with their 'non-possessive warmth'. Rogers has additionally listed some of the characteristics he considered necessary in the personality of counsellors.

(1) Social sensitivity. A person who is quite obtuse to the reactions of others, who cannot sense the ethos of an interpersonal context, who does not realize that his remarks have caused another pleasure or hurt, who does not sense friction or friendliness which exists between himself and others or between two of his acquaintances, is most unlikely to become a satisfactory counsellor.
(2) Objectivity – or controlled identification. This is not a cold detachment, but a genuinely receptive attitude and deep understanding which is not easily shocked and does not readily pass moral judgements. Yet the therapist must never get so involved with a client's

problems that he cannot provide help.

(3) Respect for individual. A person who is eager to reform students to fit his/her own standards and values is unlikely to have the capacity to respect the integrity of the student and to accept him as he is.

(4) An understanding of the self. Some counsellors have difficulty in counselling for certain problems or working with certain kinds of people. In such cases especially the counsellor needs a sound understanding through which he/she can recognize their own prejudices and the effects of their emotions on the counselling relationship. It would, therefore, seem unprofitable to choose for training those people who appear to have very rigid personality structures which may prevent them from becoming more self-aware.

(5) Psychological knowledge. A basic knowledge and understanding of human behaviour, together with its psychological social and physical determinants is an important foundation for the work of the counsellor.

Perhaps one of the most comprehensive descriptions of the 'good counsellor' can be found in a study by Kazienko and Neidt (1962) who surveyed male enrolees in 25 Counselling and Guidance Training Institutes throughout the United States. They chose as their subjects the top and bottom 25 per cent of the groups as ranked by the professional staffs of the institutes. As a result 124 counsellor trainees were placed in the 'good counsellors' category and 115 were placed in the 'poor counsellors' category. The subjects were administered the Bennett Poly-diagnostic Index in which the trainees described themselves in terms of self concept, motivating forces, feelings about others and values.

The following table lists the major self-descriptive elements that distinguished the trainees categorized as poor and those categorized as good by professional supervisors.

Poor counsellor group

Self concept – does not recognize qualities of seriousness, patience in self; loud voiced; unaware of personal self-centredness; sees self as normal, domestically, mechanically, socially and industrially minded.

Good counsellor group

Self concept – serious, earnest, patient, soft spoken; aware of personal self-centredness; more domestic than social; not mechanically or industrially minded

Motivation – Neither moved nor unmoved by prospects of security and riches.

Values – Places average value here; feels happiness lies in conformity; tends towards strict adherence to rules.

Feelings about others – Gives others no particular credit for intellectual behaviour.

Motivation – Concerned about possessing a measure of security but rejects need for wealth.

Values – Rejects cunning and shrewdness as leading to personal contentment; feels person should have right to be different; does not value severity and strictness.

Feelings about others – Views people as possessing adequate measure of ability though self-centred.

Some years ago, Farson (1954) concluded that counsellor characteristics were fundamentally those that society traditionally attributes to women; tenderness, gentleness, receptiveness and passivity. McClain (1970), too, reported that both men and women counsellors in his study appeared to possess in acceptable degree the characteristics that Farson deemed appropriate for the successful counsellor. Carkhuff and Berenson (1967) point out that recent research portrays the counsellor as not only tender, gentle and loving but also active, assertive and able to confront and interpret immediate interactions when they occur.

Inquiries into characteristics associated with counselling effectiveness (as opposed to ineffectiveness), have been approached through sociometric techniques, often with class or group members selecting from among their peers those whom they would most like to have as counsellors. Arbuckle (1956) investigated the qualities of counsellor trainees who had been selected by their classmates as individuals they would seek out when they wanted a counsellor; preferred traits were tolerance, warmth, interest, patience and sincerity. The least desirable traits were lack of understanding, lack of interest, aggressiveness, probing, moralizing, insincerity, bias, authoritarianism and a superior manner.

Communication skills

Many researchers have noted that a basic characteristic of all 'good' counsellors is an ability to communicate effectively both verbally and non-verbally. Boy and Pine (1968) have stated that effective communication occurs when the counsellor receives what the client wants to communicate, and the client receives what the counsellor wants to communicate. Communication between counsellor and client is expressed via affective, cognitive, verbal and non-verbal modes.

A counsellor needs to develop 'emotional antennae' that are keenly sensitive to the non-verbal and subtle cues conveyed through tone of voice, posture, bodily movements, a way of breathing, physical manner-isms and expressions of the eyes – in other words the subterranean signals that constitute the subliminal language of counselling.

An especially important component of effective communication is the ability to listen, the kind of listening we refer to here is completely non-evaluative. To listen the counsellor must immerse himself in the client's flow of experience and is in complete emotional and cognitive contact with the individual.

He or she should be able to sense what is going on psychologically within another person; be attuned to communications, both as receiver and sender; form balanced rational judgements while keeping himself open to feelings; be able to flexibly adapt to changing circumstances without losing identity or purpose; and, most essential of all, warmly care for the well-being of the client.

The most successful forms of treatment appear to have several things in common:

(1) Psychological change almost always occurs in a supportive, warm, empathic rewarding environment. People usually 'open up' and talk about things, and try new approaches to life, when they trust or admire or want to please the therapist. When Freud discussed the concept of the *transference relationship* he was really indicating that the client's affection for the analyst could be used to encourage the client to want to get well. When Carl Rogers wrote of the necessity for giving his clients *unconditional positive regard*, he was recognizing the power of positive reinforcement.

Encounter groups whose members focus on expressing hostility toward each other can do incredible damage – unless such expression is embedded in a background of affection and appreciation so strong that the members can tolerate occasional 'punishment' from each other. Criticism seldom cures, and too often kills all chance of improvement. Sincere expressions of warmth and tolerance for 'ab-normalities' provide the atmosphere in which change can occur.

The best forms of therapy seem to build on strengths rather than attacking weaknesses. By helping the client work towards positive improvement – toward self-actualization and good mental health –

the therapist motivates the client to continue to grow and change. Therapies that focus entirely on uncovering or discussing psychological problems may merely confirm the client's attitude that sickness is inevitable, and that he is sick.

(2) Most successful forms of treatment can be seen as feedback mechanisms. That is, they provide the client with information about what happened in the past; they put the person in touch with the functioning of his or her body; they make the individual aware of how his or her behaviour actually affects other people; they help the person realize the distance between desired goals and present achievements; or they offer information on how the social environment influences the person's thoughts, feelings and behaviours. Ideally, a complete form of therapy would do all these things – and give the client the skills to seek out and make even more effective use of feedback in the future.

THE EFFECTIVE CLIENT

The client who is most suitable for therapy has been termed the YAVIS client, i.e. young, attractive, verbal, intelligent and successful. Freud had put it more simply 'not too old, not too ill'. Predictive factors according to Luborsky et al. (1975) are:

adequacy of personality functioning; absence of schizoid trends; motivation and/or positive expectation; intelligence; initial anxiety and other strong affect like depression; educational and social assets; and 'experiencing' – rated from early psychotherapy sessions, i.e. the patient is capable of deep and immediate feelings and of being reflectively aware of these feelings.

Motivation for change is also vital, as too the willingness to be self-revealing (Malan, 1973). Low socio–economic status is negatively related to improvement in a number of American studies (Garfield, 1971). Similarly paranoid conditions are exceptionally resistant to change. Certain environmental conditions outside the therapy context produce an impossible situation for successful therapy. Clients trapped in an unresolvable marital or family problem, financial worries or physical handicap for instance may not respond to therapy unless other help, alleviating the external difficulties, can be forthcoming.

But if a person's psychological problems are construed as signs or symptoms of illness, this virtually precludes attempts to directly change the specific problem behaviour, or to directly retrain him. More importantly, if psychological problems are signs of illnesses, then the person is automatically regarded as a patient, and this process of labelling turns out to be of considerable psychological significance (e.g. Rosenhan, 1973).

CONCLUSION

All therapists agree they can help some people, but they don't all have the same people in mind and they don't share the same view of what is wrong or what constitutes help. But everybody can be helped by some therapy if appropriate expectations, goals, techniques and contexts are provided. It is not therapies as such that are ineffective. They are all designed to work, if they are properly applied. And as all of them have to be applied by the person of the therapist, it follows that, no matter what the form of treatment, for therapy to work at all the therapist must possess certain facilitating characteristics. The most significant resource any therapist brings to a helping relationship whatever his theoretical persuasion is himself. It would seem above all else that the interaction between counsellor and client is the essential factor in therapeutic change, this interaction can only develop with voluntary acceptance by each person of the other. All forms of therapy will achieve some successes but neither problems nor cures occur in a vacuum. No matter how well a patient may respond in a hospital setting, no matter what insights a client achieves in a therapist's office, the ultimate test of therapy comes when the person returns to his or her usual environment. If the client can function successfully and happily in the real world, in everyday life, we can then conclude that a 'cure' has indeed taken place.

Further reading

Arbuckle, D. S. (1956). Client perception of counsellor personality. *J. Counsel. Psychol.*, **3**, 93–6

Association for Counsellor Education and Supervision. (1964). The Counsellor, Professional Preparation Role. *Person. Guid. J.*, **42**, 536–41

Bergin, A. F. and Garfield, S. (eds.) (1971). *Handbook of Psychotherapy & Behavior Change.* (New York: John Wiley)

Rackman, S. J. and Wilson G. T. (1980). *The Effects of Psychological Therapy.* (Oxford: Pergamon)

Smale, G. (1977). *Prophecy, Behaviour & Change.* (London: Routledge & Kegan Paul)

Truax, C. B. and Carkhuff, R. R. (1967). *Towards Effective Counseling and Psychotherapy; Training and Practice.* (Chicago: Aldine)

REFERENCES

AAHP (1962). *Articles of Association*. American Association of Humanistic Psychology.

Ackerman, N. W. (1966). *Treating the Troubled Family*. (New York: Basic Books)

Allport, G. W. (1962). Psychological models for guidance. *Harvard Educ. Rev.*, **32**, 378–81

Arbuckle, D. S. (1956). Client perception of counsellor personality. *J. Counsel. Psychol.*, **3**, 93–6

Atthowe, J. and Krasner, L. (1968). A preliminary report on the application of reinforcement procedures on a chronic psychiatric ward. *J. Abnorm. Psychol.*, **73**, 37–43

Austin, L. (1948). Trends in the differential treatment in social casework. *J. Soc. Casework*, June, 203–11

Ayllon, T. and Azrin, N. (1969). *The Token Economy*. (New York: Appleton-Century-Crofts)

Bandura, A. (1965). Influence of models reinforcement contingencies on the acquisition of imitative responses. *J. Pers. Soc. Psychol.*, **1**, 589–95

Bandura, A. (1969). *Principles of Behaviour Modification*. (New York: Holt, Rinehart and Winston)

Bandura, A. (1977). *Social Learning Theory*. (New Jersey: Prentice Hall)

Bandura, A., Ross, D. and Ross, S. A. (1963). Imitation of film, mediated aggressive models. *J. Abnorm. Soc. Psychol.*, **66**, 3–11

Bandura, A., Grusec, J. and Menlove, F. (1967). Vicarious extinction of avoidance behaviour. *J. Pers. Soc. Psychol.*, **5**, 449–55

Bandura, A., Blanchard, E. and Ritter, B. (1969). The relative efficiency of desensitisation and modelling approaches for inducing behavioural, affective and cognitive changes. *J. Pers. Soc. Psychol.*, **13**, 173–99

Bandura, A., Jeffrey, R. and Wright, C. L. (1974). Efficiency of participant modeling as a function of response induction aids. *J. Abnorm. Psychol.*, **83**, 56–64

Basmajian, J. V. and Hatch, J. P. (1979). Biofeedback and modification of skeletal muscular dysfunction. In Gatehil, R. and Price, K. (eds.) *Clinical Applications of Biofeedback*. (New York: Pergamon)

Bateson, G. et al (1956). Towards a theory of schizophrenia. *Behav. Sci.*, **1**, 251–64

Beck. A. T. (1963). Thinking & Depression. *Arch. Gen. Psychiatry*, **9**, 324–33

Beck. A. T. (1976). *Cognitive Therapy & the Emotional Disorders*. (New York: International Universities Press)

Beck. A. T. *et al.* (1977). *Cognitive therapy for depression*. Upub. paper, University of Pennsylvania

Becker, N., Madsen, C., Arnold, R. and Thomas, D. (1976). The contingent use of teacher attention and praise in reducing classroom behaviour problems. *J. Spec. Educ.*, **1**, 287–307

Beers, C. (1908). *A Mind that Found Itself.* (New York: Doubleday)

Bergin, A. E. (1975). Individual psychotherapy. In Rosenzweig, M. and Porter, L. (eds.) *Annual Review of Psychology.* (Palo Alto: Ann. Rev. Inc.)

Berne, E. (1964). *Games People Play.* (New York: Grove Press)

Berne, E. (1966). *Principles of Group Treatment.* (New York: Oxford University Press)

Berne, E. (1972). *What do You Say After You Say Hello.* (London: Corgi Books)

Binswanger, L. (1955). *Ausgenwählte Vortrage und Aufsätze. Vol. 2.* (Berne: University of Berne)

Blackman, D. E. (1973). The growing impact of behavioural technology. Paper given to Section J, *Br. Assoc. Advanc. Sci.*

Blakemore, C. B. and Thorpe, J. G. (1963). The application of paradic aversion conditioning in a case of transvestism. *Behav. Res. Ther.*, **1**, 29–34

Blanchard, E. and Young L. (1974). Of promises and evidence. *Psychol. Bull.*, **81**, 44–6

Boss, M. (1957). Daseinanalysis. In Masserman, J. and Moreno, J. (eds.) *Progress in Psychotherapy.* (New York: Grune & Stratton)

Boy, A. V. and Pine, G. J. (1968). *The Counsellor in the Schools.* (New York: Houghton Mifflin)

Brammer, L. M. and Shostrom, E. L. (1964). *Therapeutic Psychology.* (Englewood Cliffs: Prentice Hall)

Brown, G. W., Birley, J. L. and Wine, J. K. (1972). Influence of family life on the course of schizophrenic disorders. *Br. J. Psychiatry*, **121**, 242–58

Bruner, J. S. and Goodman, C. (1947). Value and need as organising factors in perception. *J. Abnorm. Soc. Psychol.*, **42**, 33–44

Burns, R. B. (1979). *The Self Concept.* (Harlow: Longmans)

Burns, R. B. (1982). *Self Concept Development and Education.* (London: Holt, Rinehart and Winston)

Butler, J. M. and Haigh, G. V. (1954). Changes in the relation between self concept and ideal concepts consequent upon client centered counseling. In Rogers, C. R. and Dymond, R. F. (eds.) *Psychotherapy & Personality Change.* pp. 55–75. (Chicago: University of Chicago Press)

Camus, A. (1955). *The Myth of Sisyphus and other Essays.* (New York: Random House)

Carkhuff, R. (1969). *Helping & Human Relations.* (New York: Holt, Rinehart and Winston)

Carkhuff, F. and Berenson, B. (1967). *Beyond Counseling and Therapy.* (New York: Holt, Rinehart and Winston)

Carney, A. *et al.* (1978). The combination of hormonal & psychological treatment for female sexual unresponsiveness. *Br. J. Psychiatry*, **133**, 339–46

Cautela, J. (1967). Covert sensitisation. *Psychol. Rep.*, **20**, 459–68

Cawley, R. H. (1977). *The Teaching of Psychotherapy.* Association of University Teachers of Psychiatry. (Newsletter.) January. 19–36

Chesler, P. (1972). *Women & Madness.* (New York: Doubleday)

Chomsky, N. (1972). Psychology and ideology. *Cognition*, **1**, 11–46

Cullen. C., Hattersley, J. and Tennant, L. (1977). Behaviour modification – some implications of a radical behaviourist view. *Bull. Br. Psychol. Soc.*, **30**, 65–8

Davey, G. (1981). How Skinner's theories work. *Bull. Br. Psychol. Soc.*, **34**, 57–60

Davison, G. C. (1976). Homosexuality: the ethical challenge. *J. Consult. Clin. Psychol.*, **44**, 157–62

Dinkmeyer, D. and Muro, J. (1971). *Group Counseling: Theory & Practice.* (New York: Peacock)

Dollard, J. and Miller, N. E. (1950). *Personality & Psychotherapy.* (New York: McGraw Hill)

Dominian, J. (1972). Marital pathology. *Postgrad. Med. J.*, **48**, 517–25

Ellis, A. (1958). Rational psychotherapy. *J. Gen. Psychol.*, **59**, 35–49

Ellis, A. (1970). *The Essence of Rational Psychotherapy.* (New York: Institute for Rational Living)

Ellis, A. (1977). Rational–emotive therapy. *Counsell. Psycholog.*, **7**, 2–24

Engel, B. T. (1972). Operant conditioning of cardiac function: a status report. *Psychophysiology*, **9**, 161–77

English, H. B. and English, A. C. (1958). *A Comprehensive Dictionary of Psychological and Psychoanalytic Terms.* (New York: McKay)

Eysenck, H. J. (1952). The effects of psychotherapy: an evaluation. *J. Consult. Psychol.*, **16**, 319–24

Eysenck, H. J. (1955). The effects of psychotherapy: a reply. *J. Abnorm. Soc. Psychol.*, **50**, 147–8

Fagan, J. (1970). The task of the therapist. In Fagan, J. and Shepard, I. (eds.) *Gestalt Therapy Now.* (New York: Science and Behaviour Books)

Fairweather, G. W. (1964). *Social Psychology in treating Mental Illness.* (New York: John Wiley)

Fairweather, G. W. and Simon, R. (1963). A further follow up comparison of psychotherapeutic programs. *J. Consult. Psychol.*, **27**, 186

Farson, R. E. (1954). The counsellor is a woman. *J. Counsell. Psychol.*, **1**, 221–3

Feldman, M. P. and Macculloch, M. J. (1965). The application of anticipatory avoidance learning in the treatment of homosexuality. *Behav. Res. Ther.*, **2**, 165–83

Fiedler, R. E. (1950). A comparison of therapeutic relations in psychoanalytic, non-directive, and Adlerian therapy. *J. Consult. Psychol.*, **14**, 436–56

Foreyt, J. and Kennedy, W. (1971). Treatment of overweight by aversion therapy. *Behav. Res. Ther.*, **9**, 29–34

Foxx, R. and Azrin, N. (1973). *Toilet Training the Retarded.* (Champaigne, Ill: Research Press)

Frank, J. D. (1968). The influence of patients' and therapists' expectations on the outcome of psychotherapy. *Br. J. Med. Psychol.*, **41**, 349–56

Frank, J. D. (1977). The two faces of psychotherapy. *J. Nerv. Ment. Dis.*, **164**, 3–7

Franks, C. M. and Wilson, G. T. (1975). *Annual Review of Behavior Therapy.* Vol. III. (New York: Brunner Mazel)

Freud, A. (1936). *The Ego and the Mechanisms of Defence.* (London: Hogarth Press)

Freud, S. (1900). *The Interpretation of Dreams*. (Standard Ed.), Vols. 4 & 5. (London: Hogarth Press)

Freud, S. (1901). *The Psychopathology of Everyday Life*. (Standard Ed.), Vol. 6. (London: Hogarth Press)

Freud, S. (1905). *Analysis of a Phobia in a Five Year Old Boy*. (Standard Ed.), Vol. 10. (London: Hogarth Press)

Freud, S. (1913). *On Beginning the Treatment*. (Standard Ed.), Vol. 12. (London: Hogarth Press)

Freud, S. (1926). *Inhibitions, Symptoms & Anxiety*. (Standard Ed.), Vol. 20. (London: Hogarth Press)

Freud, S. (1933). *New Introductory Lectures*. (Standard Ed.), Vol. 22. (London: Hogarth Press)

Freud, S. (1937). *Analysis Terminable and Interminable*. (Standard Ed.), Vol. 23. (London: Hogarth Press)

Garfield, S. L. and Bergin, A. (1978). *Handbook of Psychotherapy & Behavior Change*. (New York: John Wiley)

Garfinkel, P. E., Kline, S. A. and Stancer, H. (1973). Treatment of anorexia nervosa using operant conditioning. *J. Nerv. Mental. Dis.*, **157**, 428–33

Garvey, W. P. and Hegrenes, J. R. (1966). Desensitization techniques in the treatment of school phobia. *Am. J. Orthopsychiatry*, **36**, 147–52

Goldfried, M. and Davison, G. C. (1976). *Clinical Behavior Therapy*. (New York: Holt, Rinehart and Winston)

Gomez-Schwartz, B. *et al.* (1978). Individual psychotherapy & behavior therapy. In Rosenzweig, M. and Porter, L. (eds.) (Palo Alto: Ann. Rev. Inc.)

Greening, T. (1977). The Gestalt Prayer: final version? *J. Humanist. Psychol.*, **17**, 127–9

Greenspoon, J. (1955). The reinforcing effect of two spoken sounds on the frequency of two responses. *Am. J. Psychol.*, **68**, 409–16

Grunbaum, A. (1977). How scientific is psychoanalysis. In Stern, R. (ed.) *Science & Psychotherapy*. (New York: Haven Press)

Halmos, P. (1965). *The Faith of the Counsellors*. (London: Constable)

Hanley, D. (1971). The effects of short term counselling. *Dissertation Abst.*, **31**, 5126–27

Harris, T. (1967). *I'm OK – You're OK*. (New York: Harper Row)

Heidegger, M. (1949). *Existence & Being*. (Chicago: Regnery Press)

Hilgard, E. and Bower, J. (1975). *Theories of Learning*. (Englewood Cliffs: Prentice Hall)

Hogan, R. A. and Kirchner, J. H. (1967). Preliminary report of the extinction of learned fears via implosive therapy. *J. Abnorm. Psychol.*, **72**, 106–109

Horney, K. (1950). *Neurosis & Human Growth*. (New York: Norton)

Hunziker, J. C. (1972). The use of participant modelling in the treatment of water phobia. *Masters Thesis*. Arizona State University

Janda, L. and Rimm, D. C. (1972). Covert sensitization in the treatment of obesity. *J. Abnorm. Psychol.*, **80**, 37–42

Janov, A. (1970). *The Primal Scream*. (New York: Dell Publishing)

Jones, M. (1952). *Social Psychiatry*. (London: Tavistock Press)

Jones, M. C. (1924). A laboratory study of fear. *Pedagog. Sem.*, **31**, 308–15

Jung, C. G. (1960). The Structure & Dynamics of the Psyche. *The Collected Works of Jung*. Vol. 8. (London: Routledge & Kegan Paul)

Kazdin, A. and Bootzin, R. (1972). The token economy. *J. Appl. Behav. Anal.*, **5**, 343–72

Kazdin, A. and Wilcoxon, L. (1976). Systematic desensitisation & non-specific treatment effects. *Psychol. Bull.*, **83**, 729–58

Kazdin, A. and Wilson, G. T. (1978). Criteria for evaluating psychotherapy. *Arch. Gen. Psychiatry*, **35**, 407–18

Kazienko, L. W. and Neidt, C. (1962). Self descriptions of good & bad counsellor trainees. *Counsellor Educ. Superv.*, **1**, 100–23

Kempler, W. (1973). Gestalt therapy. In Corsini, R. (ed.) *Current Psychotherapies*. (Itasca: Peacock)

Kierkegaard, S. A. (1954). *The Sickness unto Death*. (New York: Doubleday)

Klein, M. (1932). *The Psychoanalysis of Children*. (London: Hogarth Press)

Kline, P. (1972). *Fact & Fantasy in Freudian Theory*. (London: Methuen)

Koestler, A. (1967). *The Ghost in the Machine*. (London: Hutchinson)

Kovel, J. (1976). *A Complete Guide to Therapy*. (New York: Pantheon)

Krasner, L. (1969). Behaviour modification values and training. In Franks, C. (ed.) *Behaviour Therapy*. (New York: McGraw Hill)

Kravetz, R. and Forness, S. (1971). The classroom as a desensitising setting. *Except. Child.*, **37**, 389–91

Laing, R. D. (1967). *The Politics of Experience*. (New York: Pantheon)

Laing, R. D. and Esterson, A. (1964). *Sanity, Madness & the Family*. (London: Tavistock Press)

Lake, F. (1978). Treating psychosomatic disorders related to birth trauma. *J. Psychosom. Res.*, **30**, 6–11

Lambert, M., Segger, J., Staley, J. and Spenser, B. (1978). Reported self concept and self actualising value changes as a function of academic classes with wilderness experience. *Percept. Mot. Skills.*, **46**, 1035–40

Lange, A. and Jakubowski, P. (1976). *Responsible Assertive Behavior*. (Champaigne: Research Press)

LaPointe, K. and Harrel, T. (1978). Thoughts and feelings. *Cognit. Ther. Res.*, **2**, 311–22

Lazarus, A. A. (1963). The results of behaviour therapy in 126 cases of severe neurosis. *Behav. Res. Ther.*, **1**, 65–78

Leboyer, F. (1977). *Birth Without Violence*. (London: Fontana)

Leung, F. (1975). The ethics and scope of behaviour modification. *Bull. Br. Psychol. Assoc.*, **28**, 376–79

Levine, F. and Fasnacht, G. (1974). Token rewards may lead to token learning. *Am. Psychol.*, **29**, 816–20

Levinger, G. (1966). Sources of marital disatisfaction among applicants for divorce. *Am. J. Orthopsychiatry*, **36**, 803–7

Levitsky, A and Perls, F. (1970). The rules and games of Gestalt therapy. In Fagan, J. and Shepherd, I. (eds.) *Gestalt Therapy Now*. (Palo Alto: Science and Behaviour Books)

Levitsky, A. and Perls, F. (1972). The rules and games of Gestalt Therapy. In Huber, J. and Millman, L. (eds.) *Goals and Behaviour in Psychotherapy and Counseling*. (Columbus, Ohio: Merrill)

Liberman, R. (1970). Behaviourist approaches to family and couple therapy. *Am. J. Orthopsychiatry*, **40**, 106–18

Lichtenstein, E. *et al.* (1973). Comparison of rapid smoking, warm smoky air and attention placebo in the modification of smoking behavior. *J. Consult. Clin. Psychol.*, **40**, 92–8

Lieberman, M. A., Miles, M. B. and Yalom, I. D. (1973). *Encounter Groups: First Facts.* (New York: Basic Books)

Liebert, R. and Spiegler, M. (1974). *Personality. Strategies for the Study of Man*, (Homewood: Dorsey Press)

London, P. (1972). The end of ideology in behavior modification. *Am. Psychol.*, **27**, 913–20

Lovaas, O. I. (1966). A programme for the establishment of speech in children. In King, J. W. (ed.) *Early Childhood Autism.* (New York: Pergamon)

Luborsky, L. *et al.* (1975). Comparative studies of psychotherapies. *Archiv. Gen. Psychiatry*, **32**, 995–1008

Luria, H. (1961). *The Role of Speech in the Regulation of Normal and Abnormal Behavior.* (New York: Liveright Press)

Luria, Z. (1959). A semantic analysis of a normal and a neurotic therapy group. *J. Abnorm. Soc. Psychol.*, **58**, 216–20

McClain, E. (1970). Personal growth of teachers in training through self study. *J. Teacher Educ.*, **21**, 372–7

Mackinnon, D. and Dukes, W. (1962). Regression. In Portman, L. (ed.) *Psychology in the Making.* (New York: Knopf)

Mahler. C. A. (1969). *Group Counseling in Schools.* (New York: Houghton Mifflin)

Malan, D. H. (1973). The outcome problem in psychotherapy research. *Arch. Gen. Psychiatry*, **29**, 719–29

Marks, I. M. and Gelder, M. G. (1965). A controlled retrospective study of behaviour therapy in phobic patients. *Br. J. Psychiatry*, **111**, 561–73

Marzagao, L. (1972). Systematic desensitisation treatment of kleptomania, *J. Behav. Ther. Exp. Psychiatry*, **3**, 327–28

Masters, W. H. and Johnson, V. E. (1966). *Human Sexual Response.* (Boston: Little, Brown)

Masters, W. H. and Johnson, V. E. (1970). *Human Sexual Inadequacy.* (London: Churchill)

Mathews, A. *et al.* (1976). Imaginal flooding and exposure to real phobic situations. *Br. J. Psychiatry*, **129**, 362–71

May, J. R. (1977). Psychophysiology of self-regulated phobic thoughts. *Behav. Ther.*, **8**, 150–9

May, R. *et al.* (1958). *Existence: A New Dimension in Psychiatry and Psychology.* (New York: Basic Books)

Mead, G. H. (1934). *Mind, Self and Society.* (Chicago: University of Chicago Press)

Meichenbaum, D. (1977). *Cognitive Behavior Modification.* (New York: Plenum Press)

Melamed, B. G. (1977). Psychological preparation for hospitalisation. In Rachman, S. (ed.) *Contributions to Medical Psychology.* (London: Pergamon)

Meyer, A. J. and Henderson, J. B. (1974). Multiple risk factor reduction in the prevention of cardiovascular disease. *Prevent. Med.*, **3**, 225–36

Meyer, V. and Chesser, E. (1970). *Behaviour Therapy in Clinical Psychiatry.* (Harmondsworth: Penguin)

Miller, N. E. (1969). Learning of visceral and glandular responses. *Science*, **163**, 434–5

Miller, N. E. (1972). Interaction between learned and physical factors in mental illness. *Semin. Psychiatry*, **4**, 239–54

Miron, N. B. (1968). Issues and implications of operant conditioning. *Hosp. Community Psychiatry*, **19**, 226–8

Mitchell, K. *et al.* (1977). A reappraisal of the therapeutic effectiveness of accurate empathy, nonpossessive warmth and genuineness. In Gurman, A. and Razin, A. (eds.) *Effective Psychotherapy.* (Oxford: Pergamon)

Mowrer, O. H. (1964). *The New Group Therapy.* (New Jersey: Van Nostrand Reinhold)

Nelson-Jones, R. (1982). *The Theory and Practice of Counselling Psychology.* (London: Holt, Rinehart and Winston)

Orme, M. and Purnell, R. (1968). Behaviour modification and transfer in and out of control classroom. Presented to *Am. Educ. Res. Assoc.*, Chicago

Orwell, G. (1954). *Nineteen Eighty Four.* (Harmondsworth: Penguin)

Parrino, J. (1971). Reduction of seizures by desensitization. *J. Behav. Ther. Exp. Psychiatry*, **2**, 215–18

Patterson, C. (1973). *Theories of Counseling and Psychotherapy.* (New York: Harper & Row)

Patterson, C. (1977). New approaches in counselling. *Br. J. Guidance Counsell.*, **5**, 9–15

Paul, G. L. and Bernstein, D. (1973). *Anxiety and Clinical Problems.* (Morristown, NJ: General Learning Press)

Perls, F. (1969). *Gestalt Therapy Verbatim.* (Lafayette: Real People Press)

Rachlin, H. (1976). *Behavior and Learning.* (San Francisco: W. H. Freeman)

Rachman, S. (1966a). Sexual fetishism. *Psychol. Rec.*, **16**, 293–6

Rachman, S. (1966b). Studies in desensitization. *Behav. Res. Ther.*, **4**, 1–6

Rachman, S. J. and Wilson, G. T. (1980). *The Effects of Psychological Therapy*, 2nd Edn. (Oxford: Pergamon)

Rank, O. (1929). *The Trauma of Birth.* (London: Routledge & Kegan Paul)

Rimm, D., Hill, G., Brown, N. and Suart, J. (1974). Group assertive training in the treatment of expression of inappropriate anger. *Psychol. Rep.*, **84**, 791–98

Rimm, D. C. and Litvak, S. B. (1969). Self verbalisation and emotional arousal. *J. Abnorm. Psychol.*, **32**, 564–74

Rimm, D. C. and Masters, J. C. (1974). *Behavior Therapy.* (New York: Academic Press)

Rimm, D. and Medeiros, D. (1970). The role of muscle relaxation in participant modelling. *Behav. Res. Ther.*, **8**, 127–32

Rogers, C. R. (1947). Current trends in psychotherapy. In Dennis, W. (ed.) *Current Trends in Psychotherapy.* (Pittsburgh: University of Pittsburgh)

Rogers, C. R. (1951). *Client Centred Therapy.* (Boston: Houghton Mifflin)

Rogers, C. R. (1956). Intellectualised psychotherapy. *Contemp. Psychol.*, **1**, 357–8

Rogers, C R. (1957). The necessary and sufficient conditions of therapeutic personality change. *J. Consult. Psychol.*, **21**, 95–103

Rogers, C. R. (1959). A theory of therapy, personality and interpersonal relationships as developed in the client-centered framework. In Koch, S. (ed.) *Psychology: a Study of a Science.* Vol. 3, 184–256. (New York: McGraw Hill)

Rogers, C. R. (1961). *On Becoming a Person.* (Boston: Houghton Mifflin)

Rogers, C. R. (1967). Towards a modern approach to values. In Rogers, C. R. and Stephens, B. (eds.) *Person to Person.* (London: Souvenir Press)

Rogers, C. R. (1969). *Freedom to Learn.* (Columbus, Ohio: Merrill)

Rogers, C. R. (1970). *Encounter Groups.* (New York: Harper Row)

Rogers, C. R. (1974). In Retrospect. *Amer. Psychol.*, **29**, 115

Rogers, C. R. and Dymond, R. F. (1954). *Psychotherapy and Personality Change.* (Chicago: University of Chicago Press)

Rogers, C. R., Gendlin, E. T., Kiesler, D. and Truax, C. (1967). *The Therapeutic Relationship and its Impact.* (Madison: University of Wisconsin Press)

Rogers, T. and Craighead, W. (1977). Physiological responses to self-statements. *Cognit. Ther. Res.*, **1**, 99–120

Sanderson, R., Campbell, D. and Laverty, S. (1963). Traumatically conditioned responses acquired during respiratory paralysis. *Nature*, **196**, 1235–6

Sanford, N. (1954). Clinical methods: Psychotherapy. *Ann. Rev. Psychol.*, **5**, 311–16

de Sharmes, R. *et al.* (1954). A note on attempted evaluations of psychotherapy. *J. Clin. Psychol.*, **10**, 233–5

Sherman, A. R. (1973). *Behaviour Modification.* (Monterey: Brooks Cole)

Shertzer, B. and Stone, S. (1976). *Fundamentals of Guidance.* (Boston: Houghton Mifflin)

Shlien, J., Mosak, H, and Dreikurs, R. (1962). Effects of time limits. *J. Counsel. Psychol.*, **9**, 31–4

Shoben, E. J. (1949). Psychotherapy as a problem in learning theory. *Psychol. Bull.*, **46**, 366–92

Skinner, B. F. (1951). How to teach animals. *Scient. Am.*, **185**, 26–9

Skinner, B. F. (1971). *Beyond Freedom & Dignity.* (New York: Knopf)

Skynner, A. C. R. (1976). *One Flesh: Separate Persons.* (London: Constable)

Sloane, R. B. *et al.* (1975). *Psychotherapy versus Behavior Therapy.* (Cambridge, Mass: Harvard University Press)

Smith, M. L. and Glass, C. V. (1977). Meta-analysis of psychotherapy outcome studies. *Am. Psychol.*, **32**, 752–60

Snygg, D. and Combs, A. N. (1949). *Individual Behavior: A New Frame of Reference for Psychology.* (New York: Harper & Row)

Speck, R. and Attneave, C. (1973). *Family Networks.* (New York: Pantheon)

Stampfl, T. and Levis, D. (1967). Essentials of implosive therapy. *J. Abnorm. Psychol.*, **72**, 496–503

Sterman, M. B. and Friar, L. (1972). Modifying abnormal electrical activity in epileptic patients. *Electroencephalog. Neurophysiol.*, **33**

Stevenson, W. (1953). *The Study of Behavior: Q-Technique and its Methodology.* (Chicago: University of Chicago Press)

Sylvester, J. D. and Liversedge, L. A. (1960). Conditioning and the occupational cramps. In Eysenck, H. J. (ed.) *Behaviour Therapy and the Neurosis.*

(Oxford: Pergamon)

Szasz, T. S. (1960). *The Myth of Mental Illness*. (New York: Harper)

Szasz, T. S. (1961). The uses of naming and the origin of the myth of mental illness. *Amer. Psychol.*, **16**, 59–65

Teuber, N. and Powers, E. (1953). Evaluating theory in a delinquency prevention program. *Proc. Assoc. Nerv. Ment. Dis.*, **3**, 138–47

Tobin, S. A. (1971). Saying goodbye in gestalt therapy. *Psychotherapy: Theory, Research & Practice*, **8**, 150–5

Truax, C. B. (1968). Effective ingredients in psychotherapy. *J. Counsel. Psychol.*, **10**, 256–63

Truax, C. B. and Carkhuff, R. (1967). *Towards Effective Counseling & Psychotherapy*. (Chicago: Aldine)

Truax, C. B. and Mitchell, K. (1971). Research on certain therapist interpersonal skills. In Bergin, A. and Garfield, S. (eds.) *Handbook of Psychotherapy & Behaviour Change*. (New York: John Wiley)

Tyler, L. E. (1969). *The Work of the Counselor*. (New York: Appleton-Century-Crofts)

Ullman, L. P. (1969). Behaviour therapy as social movement. In Franks, C. (ed.) *Behavior Therapy*. (New York: McGraw Hill)

Ullman, L. R., Krasner, L. and Edinger, R. (1964). Verbal conditioning of common associations in long term schizophrenic patients. *Behav. Res. Ther.*, **2**, 15–18

Vance, F. and Volsky, T. (1962). Counseling & psychotherapy: split personality or Siamese twins. *Am. Psychol.*, **17**, 564–70

Voegtlin, W. L. *et al.* (1942). Conditioned reflex therapy of chronic alcoholism *Q. J. Stud. Alcohol*, **2**, 505–11

Watson, J. B. (1924). *Behaviorism*. (New York: Norton)

Watson, J. B. and Raynor, R. (1920). Conditioned emotional reactions. *J. Exp. Psychol.*, **3**, 1–4

Wexler, D. B. (1973). Tokens and taboo. *Behaviorism*, **1**, 1–24

Wolberg, L. R. (1954). *Short Term Psychotherapy*. (New York: Grune & Stratton)

Wolpe, J. (1958). *Psychotherapy by Reciprocal Inhibition*. (Stanford: Stanford University Press)

Wolpe, J. (1969). *The Practice of Behaviour Therapy*. (Oxford: Pergamon)

Wolpe, J. and Rachman, S. (1960). Psychoanalytic evidence: a critique based on Frind's case of little Hans. *J. Nerv. Ment. Dis.*, **131**, 135–45

Wolpin, M. and Raines, J. (1966). Visual imagery, expected roles & extinction as possible factors in reducing fear and avoidance behavior. *Behav. Res. Ther.*, **4**, 25–37

Wylie, R. (1961). *The Self Concept*. (Lincoln: University of Nebraska Press)

Wylie, R. (1968). The present status of the self theory. In Borgatta & Lambert, (eds.) *Handbook on Personality*. Ch 12. (Chicago: Rand McNally)

Wylie, R. (1974). *The Self Concept. Vol. I. A Review of Methodological Considerations and Measuring Instruments (Rev. ed)*. (Lincoln: University of Nebraska Press)

Wylie, R. (1979). *The Self Concept. Vol. 2*. (Lincoln: University of Nebraska Press)

Yalom, I. D. and Lieberman, M. (1972). A study of Encounter group casualties. In Sagar, C. and Caplan, H. (eds.) *Progress in Group and Family Therapy*. (New York: Harper & Row)

Yates, A. (1975). *Theory & Practice in Behavior Therapy*. (New York: John Wiley)

INDEX